Heart
Health
for Black Women

Heart Health

for Black Women

A Natural Approach to Healing and Preventing Heart Disease

DR. BEVERLY YATES

Marlowe & Company
New York

Published by
Marlowe & Company
841 Broadway, 4th Floor
New York, NY 10003

Editor: Krista Lyons-Gould
Copy Editors: Shannon L. Donovan, Jean Blomquist
Production: Marie J. T. Vigil, Scott Fowler
Design: Marie J. T. Vigil, Scott Fowler
Cover design: Scott Fowler
Printing: Publishers Press

The information in this book is intended to help readers make informed decisions about their health and the health of their loved ones. It is not intended to be a substitute for treatment by or the advice and care of a professional health care provider. While the author and publisher have endeavored to ensure that the information presented is accurate and up to date, they are not responsible for adverse effects or consequences sustained by any person using this book.

Library of Congress Cataloging-in-Publication Data

Yates, Beverly.
  Heart health for Black women : a natural approach to healing and preventing heart disease / Beverly Yates.
     p. cm.
  Includes bibliographical references and index.
  ISBN 1-56924-619-X
    1. Heart diseases in women. 2. Heart diseases in women--Alternative treatment. 3. Women, Black--Health and hygiene. 4. Naturopathy. I. Title.

RC682 . Y38 2000
616.1'2'0082--dc21

                                                          99-051304

9 8 7 6 5 4 3 2 1
Printed in the United States of America
Distributed by Publishers Group West

Dedication

This book is dedicated to my dear mom, Mary Y. Holcombe.
You always did what was right, whether or not it was convenient.

Acknowledgments

In my life, I have many things to be grateful for. In regard to the creation of this book, I thank my mom, Mary Y. Holcombe, and my aunt, Elsie McPierce, for their ongoing review of various sections and their continuous, enthusiastic encouragement of me in doing this project. Thanks to my mother-in-law, Juanita Gonzalez, for her feedback on the rough draft. I appreciate the support and focus of my editor, Krista Lyons-Gould, whose concise and insightful commentary helped me give broader voice and added emotional depth to the wisdom I wanted to share with my readers. Thank you and many hugs to my colleague Deborah A. Carter, N.D., of the Shoals Natural Health Care Center in Muscle Shoals, Alabama, as she championed both this topic and me as a writer. Her comments during the review process kept me on track with what needed to be said. Lots of hugs and kisses to my husband, John Gonzalez, for helping to provide an oasis of calm in our home so I could write, for reviewing the manuscript at various stages, and for his unshakable confidence in me and his loving encouragement. A huge thank you to my patients for their understanding and support when I cut back my hours in the clinic and my availability to them so I could write this book. A friendly nod and thanks to the acquisitions editor, Cassandra Conyers, for calling my attention to this topic and for her help in developing the book's outline. Thank you to Thomas Thoms of the National Heart, Lung, and Blood Institute for his fast response to my request for statistical information early in this project.

I thank God for my robust health, stamina, and ability to concentrate. Without that combination, this book might not have been produced in the midst of a busy private practice in natural medicine.

Contents

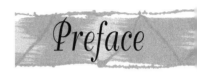

Preface

My health consciousness was raised in college, where I was first introduced to nutrition, especially macrobiotics. My love of and interest in herbs and botanical medicine grew steadily in my twenties, and I started studying with herbalists, taking classes, going to herbal retreats and workshops to learn more about medicine from the earth and how plants can serve as both food and medicine. As I observed things like watersheds and the cycle of nature firsthand, from birth to death, I came to appreciate that there are many paths to wellness. Some paths are more direct than others, yet all offer some benefits when appropriately used in the service of health restoration and wellness promotion.

I knew my maternal grandmother had an interest in herbs and used them. One was horehound (*Marrubium vulgare*), used for coughs and respiratory troubles. I remember well when Grandmom would reach for her horehound lozenges to soothe a troublesome cough. Much to my surprise and delight, I found out, when I reconnected with my father's side of the family, that my paternal great-grandmother was a medicine woman and the whole family had relied on her herbal knowledge for their health through the years. I had the good fortune to get a double dose of interest in herbs and skill with natural medicines from both sides of my family. I feel twice blessed by my ancestors and now know how this city kid came to have such a strong attraction to botanical medicine and natural approaches to health.

My family's interest in natural healing would become important later in my professional life, but after college I began working as an electrical engineer and in sales. Eventually I found myself drawn in another direction.

My decision to leave electrical engineering and sales and return to graduate school to become a naturopathic physician was a life-changing event for both my husband, John, and me. I learned about the elements of outstanding health in the physical, mental, emotional, and spiritual realms, and I happily shared that knowledge with my lifemate. (Many thanks to my husband for his willingness to share some of his recipes for your use in chapter 4. We hope you enjoy them. We also encourage you to experiment with your own variations on sweet potatoes and yams, black-eyed peas, and other traditional soul food favorites.) I would now like to share some of what I've learned with you.

African American women want true well-being as much as any other group of people. The background that we bring with us in this quest may be different than that of a man or other groups of women because some of the cultural and societal factors that influence our lives are specific to us as a group. For us or our health care practitioners to ignore the impact of these elements means we're neglecting vital clues to our health and jeopardizing our overall goal of well-being and possibly never even realizing it.

As you'll see in this book, I'm results-oriented. I'm interested in the overall "bottom line" of whether or not you have the level of health that you want. Do you?

This book is an honest, open discussion about heart health. Some of the issues I discuss came up repeatedly whenever I told people that I was writing a book on Black women and heart health. Some people thought that it was way too narrow a topic. Some expressed shock that heart disease affects Black women differently than it affects other people. Particularly enlightening was the response by doctors and physicians of all kinds, whom I was initially hopeful might be more savvy about this topic. Truly surprising were the accusations that I was racist for writing this book. The most heartening response by far was from Black women, who completely confirmed the need for this book. Without exception, all the Black women I told about this book were excited about it and pleased to know that this resource would be available. They had specific questions and concerns about heart health, as well as lots to share that was both inspiring and a continuing cause for concern.

I think every Black woman should read this book. There are so many common misperceptions around the topic of heart health, especially as it affects African American women today. Here are some of the issues and misperceptions that came up when I told a wide variety of people that I was writing this book:

All human beings need fresh air, pure water, quality food, and lots of love. In this, as people living on planet Earth, we are all the same. On that much we can agree. However, the factors that cause illness do not affect all people in exactly the same way. Just as we are not the same in how we respond to something as simple as an insult, we are not the same in our response to the factors that cause illness. Two simple examples illustrate the truth of that statement.

Five people can be together in a group when someone else hurls an insult their way. It is very likely there will be five different responses to exactly the same event. One person may be deeply offended, someone else may laugh it off right away, another person may want to turn the insult back on the offender, someone else may have hardly any response, and yet another person may decide to start a verbal self-defense class as a result of this interaction. Now, were all five people exposed to the same event? Yes. Did they all have the same response? No. Does that mean that the event has the same meaning to all the people involved? No. Are any assumptions valid here? No.

Five people may be exposed to someone with a cold who coughs and sneezes without covering their mouth or nose. These people may also be in a building or bus that has recirculated air and the air conditioning filters haven't been changed in years, if ever. The only people who catch the cold are those who are susceptible to it, those whose immune system is vulnerable to the cold virus. It is always worth exploring who is susceptible to what illnesses and learning why these people are vulnerable. In this search for knowledge lies the seeds of useful change and necessary clues about how to prevent future problems and deal with current difficulties.

Just as the people in these examples did not all respond in the same way to the same event of receiving an insult or being exposed to a cold virus, we are not the same in how we respond to the factors that create illness. As it relates to heart disease, some groups of people seem to be more affected by the levels of fat in their blood (total cholesterol, triglycerides, and three types of cholesterol: high-density lipoprotein, low-density lipoprotein, and very-low-density lipoprotein) than by high blood pressure, salt in their food, smoking, stress, or the amount of exercise they perform. Assessing risk factors for any illness means looking at the big picture and taking into consideration all elements, both separately and in combination. Sometimes one or two elements greatly outweigh all the others, while at other times single elements don't mean much by themselves and only become significant when taken all together. It is these very differences that need to be studied, understood, and acted on.

To all the people who think it's racist to write a book focused on how heart disease affects Black women:

Racism is the systematic oppression, exclusion, and harming of a group of people based on the color of their skin. That's it. Due to racism, both on purpose and by accident, there were many gaps in our knowledge about how heart disease affected most women of color, including Black women. Due to sexism, there were many gaps in our knowledge about how heart disease affected all women and about the key differences in how heart disease affected women as opposed to men.

One can slice the demographic pie lots of ways to look for information. What really matters is asking the right questions and making useful conclusions from the answers those questions produced.

To all the people who said: "A book concerning Black women and heart disease? This is too small a segment of the market to write for, study, or offer help to. The focus and scope are too narrow."

A conservative estimate is that of the U.S. population of 260 million Americans, approximately 30 million are African Americans. A bit more than half of African Americans are female, and about 70 percent are above the age of 18 years old. That means that 11 million Americans, Black women, are directly affected by the information in this book.

Heart disease is the number one killer of all Americans, and Black women are overrepresented among the people who get the sickest and die the earliest from heart disease. Lots of needless and preventable tragedies, loss, sorrow, and grief strike the lives of Black women and their loved ones—mothers, aunts, sisters, grandmothers, friends, lovers, confidantes, artists, businesswomen, doctors, lawyers, accountants, teachers, mechanics, secretaries, managers, nurses, salespeople, construction workers, dentists, therapists, counselors, nutritionists, and lots of other roles we fulfill every day of our lives.

We count. Every one of us.

"Black people don't want to be healthy. You can't sell health to these people."

Quality of life and quantity of life: we want both.

Historically, health has not been actively and continually marketed to us. Instead, poisons and toxins of every description—cigarettes, alcohol, violence, guns, illegal drugs, high-sugar and high-fat snacks—have been actively and continually marketed to us over the years. Only recently has there been the birth of a concerted effort to market health to Blacks and specifically to Black women. Every Black woman I told about this book asked when it would be published and how they could buy a copy. There was a look of genuine surprise on the faces of these women that such a work would be available and that they as a group would be the focus. Comments such as "It's about time!", "Thank you for writing this book and thinking of us," and "How can I help?" were the most common reactions by far. I feel privileged to assist my readers in creating and enjoying better heart health. Let's get to it!

Chapter 1
Does Heart Disease *Really* Affect Black Women Differently?

Does heart disease really affect Black women differently? Yes. This question is worth asking, no matter how naive it may sound. Numerous health care colleagues—both conventional and alternative practitioners—asked me this very question when they discovered I was writing this book. In fact, it was the most frequent question posed to me. Some colleagues wanted to argue about the topic, while others requested information and enlightenment. A few colleagues realized right away that they may be overlooking something important to their patients' health and important to their roles as health care providers.

Simply being asked this question and trying to answer it reveal the assumptions many health care providers make in determining who is at risk for what, and what should be done about it.

There really *are* differences in how heart disease affects Black women. As you read this book, you'll discover that the details matter.

The Number One Killer of Black Women

Heart disease, the number one killer of Black women, is an especially serious issue for us because we are at much higher risk for the health problems that make up what I call the "unholy trio"—high blood pressure, obesity, and diabetes. I believe much of this has to do with issues of lifestyle, culture, and social habits. Black women are overrepresented among the health consequences and diseases associated with smoking, obesity, diabetes, and leading a sedentary life.

These factors conspire, with the permission of the sick person to some degree, to create illness. Many lifestyle-related issues, including eating, smoking, and exercising, are within our control. You dictate what and how much you eat. Smoking, too, is a choice. We all need to understand that steady regular physical activity pays off, but it's up to us to actually exercise on a regular basis.

The actions you take day after day determine your overall health more than the things you do every once in a while to support your well-being. Just as you wouldn't prepare to run a marathon by sitting on the couch until the night before the race and then expect to do well, you won't reverse all aspects of poor heart health overnight. It takes time to get into trouble, and it takes time to heal.

Even in this seemingly health-conscious age, many Black people remain unaware of the elements of good health. Some of us even think that good health is for someone else—it's "not our thing." Nothing could be further from the truth. Great health is for everyone. Educational background, income level, gender, skin color, or family health history does not determine who deserves great health. We all deserve excellent health! Do your part to take excellent care of yourself.

What's More Deadly?

According to numerous surveys, the diseases most feared by women are cancers of the breasts, ovaries, and uterus. Approximately 200,000 women a year die of cancer. Yet heart disease is more common and kills many more women each year. Approximately 500,000 women die of diseases of the heart and blood vessels each year. Some of the skew in emphasis and awareness has to do with the fear factor: the general public is more afraid of cancer of any kind than it is of heart disease.

Because of the persistent myth that heart disease in women is rare, for many years women did not receive the same medical workup or treatment for heart disease as men did. Numerous medical studies demonstrate that women were much less likely than men to receive aggressive therapy or dramatic intervention for heart disease.

There is a continuing need for more research on the risk factors and effectiveness of treatment in Black women with heart disease compared to women of other races and ethnicities. When heart disease in women is studied, Black women often make up less than 10 percent of the study population. Many more Black women need to participate in health-related studies so the medical research community can learn about the factors of health and illness as they relate to Black women and how these factors impact our lives. There is an overall lack of information and education in the Black community about medical research. We need to know when these studies are in progress, and the researchers need to make sure we are included in significant numbers so that helpful—possibly life-saving—knowledge can be gathered. It is time to end the ignorance that surrounds our greater severity of disease, lower rates of survival, and shorter longevity compared to women of other ethnic groups in the United States.

The current medical research demonstrates important differences in the severity and consequences of various forms of heart disease among women of different races. Black women have significantly higher rates of death and greater disease severity from strokes and heart attacks than White women do. According to the *1999 Heart and Stroke Statistical Update* from the American Heart Association, the age-adjusted death rate from coronary heart disease is nearly 72 percent higher for Black women 35–74 years of age than for White women.[1] That percentage represents a dramatic difference in the outcome of heart disease.

The more informed we are as a group, the better able we are to participate in our own health care and decisions related to it. This includes personally knowing what the warning signs of heart disease are and what to do when we think something is wrong; how to track follow-up health care; and how frequently we should seek physical exams, checkups, and other measures that serve as part of an early warning system to avoid health crises. Of course, we still need to do the easiest things, like get our blood pressure checked regularly, exercise, eat well, and keep stress at a low level. Heart disease is one area of health where an ounce of prevention is easily worth a pound of cure.

Why Recognizing Heart Disease Is Important

Knowing what heart disease is and why it matters is important. It's really quite simple. Heart disease can kill you. You could leave this world in the blink of an eye if you leave heart disease untreated. But heart disease can be prevented, and its symptoms and severity can be improved with the natural and preventive measures we'll review in this book. Good heart health can allow you to live long and live well as you age. Disease and misery are not inevitable results of the aging process.

It is up to each of us to take the best possible care of ourselves. Good health allows us to enjoy our lives. Without good health, life can be more of a struggle than is necessary. Absorb all the information you can about achieving good health so you can maximize your experience of life. A resource section is included in the appendix to provide you with additional sources of information.

Today, whether you're accessing it or not, information about achieving good health is at your fingertips, but when I was a child, it just wasn't available. I am writing about heart disease because it has had a real impact on my life. Things could have been different if my family had known more about it, and I am sure this is true for many of you as well. We really did not know about heart disease, diabetes, obesity, smoking, and other factors that can cause our good health to steadily decline over time. Like most Americans, our lack of knowledge about the factors that influence health meant that we continued to make choices that promoted disease instead of health. The importance of this information is a matter of life and death.

A Personal Journey

I remember the day well. It remains a snapshot in time for me. On a warm summer Sunday afternoon in Philadelphia, my grandmother had a stroke. As that summer day unfolded—over the course of three or four hours—it became clear that something was wrong with Grandmom. Her eyes became glassy, her face sagged on one side, she couldn't talk to us, and when my mom and aunt asked her to do simple things, she didn't respond. Seemingly in an instant, the Grandmom I loved ceased to exist as I had known her.

My mom and aunt called an ambulance, but it was too late. My grandmother died two weeks later in the intensive care unit of the hospital. In fact, the last time I saw her alive was as they put her into the ambulance and took her to the hospital. Because of my age (I was 11 at the time), I was not allowed into the intensive care unit of the hospital. The hospital policy makers thought that these parts of the hospital were not appropriate for children. In this case, they were mistaken.

Over the course of two weeks, we made daily visits to the hospital (or, in my case, the hospital lobby). My mother gave me the real story about the severity of my grandmother's condition about two days before Grandmom died. I appreciated my mother telling me the truth about the situation even though her older siblings did not agree with her desire to be honest with me. Before my mother told me the real deal, I thought that Grandmom would be home soon—any day in fact—and I wanted to ask her how she was feeling. Her two-week hospitalization was the longest time we had been apart since I was a baby. I had all sorts of things I wanted to tell her about.

As a child, I did not feel protected by the hospital policy that said I could not visit my grandmother. I remember well the many attempts my cousin and I made to try to get to the upper floors of the hospital where I was sure my grandmother was waiting for our visit, only to be discovered by the hospital security guards, returned to the lobby, and kept from visiting her. After Grandmom's death, I was really angry that I did not get to see her again while she was still alive in the hospital. It was difficult for me to reconcile at the time what had happened in those two weeks between her stroke and her death.

Although my grandmother's death from stroke was my first personal brush with heart disease, it was not to be my last.

No one in our family knew any of the warning signs of stroke when my grandmother had one. If we had, maybe we could have gotten Grandmom to the hospital before serious, irreversible damage had occurred, and she might be alive today or at least have lived longer after her stroke. Who knows? By the time my family realized something serious was wrong and got Grandmom to the hospital to get help, the damage from the stroke was extensive.

It's quite possible that Grandmom also had diabetes, probably type II (adult onset). Since she rarely went to the doctor, I can't know for sure. My grandmother had a number of the symptoms of diabetes, such as frequent thirst, frequent urination, fatigue, a pervasive sense of not feeling well, and what she called "poor circulation" in her hands and feet, especially her feet. She would say to me, "Come here, child, and hold this steady for me." Looking back, I see that diabetes may have set in years before the stroke happened, but we simply didn't know what to look for in either case.

What Is Heart Disease?

As you might imagine, without proper heart function all the cells and tissues of the body are negatively affected. Heart disease robs the body of needed oxygen and other essential nutrients, such as vitamins, amino acids, minerals, and trace minerals. There is inadequate removal of normal metabolic wastes, such as carbon dioxide, from bodily cells and tissues.

Women in general have more severe forms of heart disease since they are typically older when heart problems develop.[2] Their advanced age relative to men at the onset of heart disease partially explains why women are more likely to die from heart attacks within a few weeks after their occurrence than are men.[3]

Level of education is also a factor; the risk of death from coronary heart disease is much greater for people with lower levels of education compared to highly educated people.[4]

Some surprising statistics show the extra impact heart disease has

Biggest Factors That Cause or Contribute to Heart Disease

- high blood pressure
- obesity
- diabetes
- smoking
- sedentary lifestyle
- too much stress or lack of effective skills to cope with stress

in the lives of African Americans, especially women. While some of the numbers are grim, the future is bright, provided that the origins of heart disease are treated effectively with natural and preventive measures. If the medical community's current focus continues treating only the symptoms of heart disease without treating the causes—then these sobering statistics won't significantly change for the better.

Let's make it a goal to cut heart disease frequency and severity in Black women by 50 percent by the year 2010. Do we have a deal? We can do this by becoming more knowledgeable about the causes and prevention of heart disease and by adopting healthier lifestyles.

Following are explanations about some common elements of heart and cardiovascular disease, including a discussion about what having a particular aspect of heart disease could mean to you. I've included definitions of medical terms where appropriate. I will cover the three most common kinds of heart and cardiovascular disease: high blood pressure, heart attacks, and stroke. These cause the majority of death, disease, and suffering in the lives of Black women.

Three Types of Heart Disease

High Blood Pressure

High blood pressure, also known as hypertension, is one symptom of heart disease that affects Black women much differently—and more severely—than any other group of the U.S. population. Black women have more of both undiagnosed and untreated high blood pressure than other population groups. And get this—even if it is both diagnosed and treated, high blood pressure among Black women is more likely to remain high despite therapy. For Black women, high blood pressure is the single biggest factor in developing serious, life-threatening heart disease. Though this symptom and cause of heart disease may seem typical among people you know, it is not normal.

The term "high blood pressure" means that when the heart pumps blood, it has to do so against increased pressure or resistance. It's like having to force your way through an increasingly crowded stream of foot traffic. As the pressure goes up, it becomes harder and harder to make progress. You work harder to get to the same place, and it takes more energy to do it. The importance of this is that the heart has to work harder and harder to pump blood throughout the body.

The heart never rests. It is working all the time that you are alive. When the body and mind are at rest, the heart gets to take a rest relative to the demands placed upon it when you are active. The consequence of this is that the lower the blood pressure or resistance the heart has to work against, the easier it is for the heart to pump out blood 24 hours a day, seven days a week, year in and year out. If the heart has to work very hard all the time, as it does in the case of high blood pressure, background housekeeping tasks in the heart tissue and a relative state of rest for the heart are missing.

The current medical definition of high blood pressure is a reading greater than 140/90 mm Hg (said aloud as "140 over 90") with the person sitting and relaxed. This measurement has to be done at least three times in a row with a reading equal to or higher than 140/90 each time to establish this diagnosis. The repeated measurements are done to rule out a temporary high reading, which can occur just after the person had a stressful trip to the doctor's office. Efforts are underway to reset the numbers that represent high blood pressure to 130/85, as some health care providers believe that 140/90 may not be stringent enough.

There is also a phenomenon called "white coat hypertension," in which a patient might only have high blood pressure at the doctor's office. Frequently, health care providers who suspect this syndrome will ask patients to test their blood pressure at home or in some other neutral place. Checking blood pressure outside the doctor's office minimizes negative associations the person may have with things related to their health care, doctors, or doctors' offices, and prevents patients from being treated for a condition they do not have.

Most of the causes of hypertension can be treated with natural remedies and some common sense. High blood pressure not only contributes directly to heart disease but is a symptom or signal, if you will, that there are other underlying, indirect contributors; as such, once the cause is identified and effectively treated, the high blood pressure is likely to improve. It can gradually return to normal as the reasons for it are successfully addressed.

Causes of High Blood Pressure

- stress
- eating too much salt (for people who are negatively affected by it)
- certain prescription and over-the-counter medicines
- disorders that elevate levels of adrenal hormones, especially chronic overproduction of cortisol (nature's cortisone) by the body; this typically happens in response to perceived stress of short-term or long-term duration
- diabetes
- lack of rest
- lack of exercise
- worry
- anxiety
- lack of fulfilling relationships
- financial strain, too much debt—more month than money at the month's end

Heart Attacks

A heart attack results from the heart having a chronic lack of blood supply. The heart has its own blood vessels that deliver blood to it, such as arteries, capillaries, and veins. These blood vessels for the heart are called "coronary," as in "coronary arteries." A blockage in any of these coronary arteries that interferes with the delivery of nutrients (including oxygen) to the heart tissue and the removal of normal metabolic waste products from it, kills the affected tissue. This is also known as myocardial infarction (MI). When blockages are relatively minor, the heart compensates by developing new blood vessels to go around the blockage and restore the blood supply. With significant blockages, the heart tissue can't keep up with the need for new blood vessels, and the deficit of nutrient delivery and waste removal from heart tissue builds up over time. In this situation, the damage to the heart gradually worsens.

When a local area of the heart becomes starved of nutrients—especially oxygen—long enough, the heart attempts to compensate, and the normal rhythmic activity of the heart muscle becomes arrhythmic and uncoordinated. Severe or total blockage of an area of heart tissue causes what is commonly known as a heart attack.

Strokes

The category of stroke includes cerebrovascular accidents, thromboses (clots), hemorrhages, embolisms (clots on the move), and transient ischemic attacks (TIAs occur when there's a temporary lack of blood flow to a bodily tissue, typically the brain). What is a stroke? "Stroke" describes the series of events that occur when blood flow to an area of the body is completely stopped. It is caused by either inappropriate

Herbal Warning

Two herbs are known to raise blood pressure in certain people: licorice (herbal, not the candy; plant name: *Glycyrrhiza glabra*) and ephedra (plant name: *Ephedra sinensis*). These two herbs should be used with caution if you have high blood pressure or are susceptible to it. Check your blood pressure regularly (weekly) before you start using these herbs, and continue to monitor your blood pressure while using them to be sure that it remains safe to do so. If your blood pressure increases, stop using them. There are other herbs that are helpful for a host of ailments that do not have this risk associated with their use.

Common over-the-counter medicines for allergies and sinus congestion may contain pseudoephedrine hydrochloride, a single chemical from the Ephedra plant. Pseudoephedrine can aggravate high blood pressure too.

Causes of Heart Attacks

- stress
- high-fat diet with fats of poor quality
- high-sugar diet
- lack of relaxation and play time
- not enough time for self
- no exercise
- exercise done too hard and too long, especially with inadequate preparation
- lack of proper rest and sleep
- risk is increased if there is a history of heart attacks among blood relatives
- loneliness
- isolation
- lack of fulfilling relationships
- financial difficulties
- smoking
- diabetes
- serious heart murmurs that are signals of too much backflow of blood within the heart chambers themselves (often a sign of problems with a heart valve)

clotting of blood that gets stuck in an important part of the body such as the brain, or a leaking of blood into a tissue that cannot handle it. The clot forms a blockage and deprives the affected tissue of blood. This blockage starves the affected tissue, causing the tissue to no longer be able to do its normal job.

When this happens in the brain, a person usually shows symptoms that mean something serious is wrong. Some of those symptoms are facial droop, slurred speech, paralysis (permanent or temporary), or an abrupt behavior change. Because a stroke starves the bodily tissue that it has blocked from its normal nutrient-laden blood supply, a person loses the function that the tissue used to perform. If not treated promptly, the damage can be severe and permanent. Sometimes reha-bilitation can restore partial or full function. If a full stroke receives no treatment of any kind, most likely the damage will be permanent.

Strokes can be relatively minor in extent and damage ("silent" stroke), sometimes even escaping detection because there are no obvious symptoms or signs of damage. Facial droop, slurred speech, paralysis (permanent or temporary), or abrupt behavior change are all missing in silent strokes. These common symptoms of stroke can be leading clues for doctors and other health care givers. Without these clues, there is little reason to suspect that a stroke may have occurred.

In my experience, understandably, if a patient is diagnosed years after an apparently silent stroke, they are bound to feel misled or disap-pointed that the stroke wasn't caught at the time it happened. Unfortunately, without the indicators mentioned above, it is not likely that members of the health care team would look for stroke. In today's HMO climate, where insurance companies are reluctant to spend any more for lab work and doctor's visits than what they believe is ab-solutely necessary (that is, the bare minimum), it is even less likely that a "silent" stroke will be found in the absence of other illness or symptoms.

You Are in Charge of Your Health

As you read the causes for high blood pressure and heart attacks, you may have noticed that certain factors appear repeatedly on the lists. In fact, most of these causes of heart disease have at least one thing in common: they are preventable. That's right. Stress, diets that are high in fat and sugar, smoking, and lack of exercise are all factors you can do something about. The control is in your hands.

A key distinguishing philosophy of naturopathic medicine is to treat the causes of illness rather than mask the symptoms of disease. This is the guiding theme of this book and represents the viewpoint from which I share this information. I hope that it will stimulate your own thinking and help you to clarify your assessment of your current heart health. Ideally, you will be able to determine what—if anything—needs to change so you can create, maintain, and increase the level of heart and cardiovascular health you experience for your lifetime. It is central to your ability to enjoy both the quality of life and the quantity of life you live in a healthy, zestful manner.

---

[1] American Heart Association. *1999 Heart and Stroke Statistical Update.* (Dallas, Texas: American Heart Association, 1999), 10.

[2] Ibid., 11.

[3] Ibid.

[4] Ibid., 10.

Chapter 2
Why Heart Disease Commonly Strikes Black Women

Let's explore why heart disease is generally more deadly in women and, in particular, why it is most deadly in African American women. Many people asked me, "Why is heart disease such a problem for Black women?" as I wrote this book. The more I explained it, the more I came to realize that the typical person (of any gender, race, or ethnicity) knows very little about the factors that actually create heart health or heart disease. People most frequently ask about the roles of nutrition and exercise, thinking that those lifestyle factors alone are the source of problems. For many African American women, these are key factors, but rarely are they the only factors that determine our level of heart health.

In this chapter, we'll look at some expected and some unexpected, perhaps even controversial, aspects of lifestyle choices, habits, current cultural influences, and historical events that may all be coming together to play a part in the level of heart health experienced by African American women today. Some of what I present has extensive research to back it up. You'll also read my own speculation about what may be affecting the relative heart health of African American women, which will help to explain why we have the worst level of heart health in America at this time.

We are the only category of Americans for whom heart health statistics have worsened over the last 10 years.

Lifestyle habits like too little exercise; eating foods high in fat and sugar and low in fiber; extraordinary levels of chronic, unrelieved stress; and jobs that require us to sit still for much of the day are reversing heart health toward serious forms of heart disease. Some people are being affected more severely. Yet these habits can be changed, and to a large extent, the advice about how to deal with high blood pressure, high cholesterol, and other causes of heart disease is the same regardless of gender, race, age, or ethnicity. Aerobic exercise, excellent nutrition, and awareness of effective health habits are things we all need to pay attention to.

Heritage does not influence these kinds of lifestyle approaches to creating a healthy heart. But our heritage is linked to the reasons why heart health is a problem for us as a particular group of people.

As you'll discover in this chapter, when you examine the different factors that contribute to heart disease from a historical perspective, you can understand why Black women experience heart disease more frequently and more severely than any other group of people in the United States. Some of the relevant factors are poor nutrition, lack of exercise, stress, diabetes, doing too much for everyone else but oneself, and social compensations developed under extreme stress.

Factors That Create or Destroy the Healthy Heart

Why does heart disease strike Black women more frequently and more severely than other groups? To begin with, let's look at the tangible factors that may be leading to increased risk.

Obesity

Cultural Values from Our West African Ancestors—For the most part, we've inherited our cultural values from our West African ancestors. Numerous groups there have historically held overweight members of the community in high esteem; it meant that they had plenty to eat and was considered a sign of prosperity and wealth.

Being overweight is also associated with other symbols of health and prosperity in our collective cultural history. Fat was part of the Goddess image, a symbolic representation of a woman in all her distinctly female form, accentuating her feminine curves. These very same curves, composed primarily of a woman's breasts and hips, are where fat most readily accumulates on a typical woman's body. The Goddess was part of a rich spiritual tradition in which women were strongly associated with the power of creation, especially the power to bring other people to life through childbirth. This was considered a special and awesome power, an acknowledgment of something only women can do. Women's roles as healers in the community also played a part in the cycle of birth and death. When the Goddess was represented through art—in pictures, sketches, and sculptures—she was shown in a multitude of forms: her voluptuous form, her pregnant form, and her birth-giving form. These artistic representations express the mysticism, reverence, and power associated with the Goddess. Her accentuated fertility was symbolic of a cultural expression of wealth, abundance, and power.

In traditional West African cultures, fat women were considered beautiful; thin or slender women were not considered as physically attractive or fertile. A healthy woman who could survive multiple births could give life to others and increase the number of people available to help sustain the village, thereby increasing the communal wealth. We now know that for a woman to successfully bear children, she needs a certain level of body fat. Women with extremely low levels of body fat (such as some elite athletes and anorexics) can have a more difficult time with childbearing and risk having their menstrual cycles stop altogether.

Some of that cultural preference carries over into our lives today. African American women who are slender are often harassed for being too skinny and frequently told they need to "put some meat on them bones." While a slender girl child is often told this in a playful setting or with a playful tone of voice, she comes to realize that there is another dynamic at play in those words. It may hint at a concern for future health ("If you get sick, you won't have any weight to draw on to get you through it") or serve as a warning about future desirability as a sexual partner or eligibility for marriage.

While I do not want to romanticize the traditional and historical views of being fat, I do want to point out that there are multiple roots that make up the overall cultural bias toward acceptance of increased levels of body fat. I have noted that in the Black community, we do not look at each other as harshly about being fat as White Americans do, and there are more Black women who are fat—truly obese. Our ancestral value of fat as good is at odds with the advertising messages constantly promoted in the United States that say "thin is in," even though those body images are unrealistic for most women of any race or ethnicity. Less than two percent of the female population has the body type favored by the fashion and cosmetics industries. But as more African Americans experience economic affluence, it appears that our attitudes about obesity and being fat are shifting. More Black women are experiencing discrimination and social stigma for being fat. These shifting attitudes and perceptions about fat may have more to do with issues of economic class than race.

What's Being Fat Got to Do with It?—As a group, Black women are the most overweight segment of the U.S. population. Recent studies have reported that over 50 percent of Black women in the United States are obese. Heart disease is more common among people who are overweight or obese. Being overweight or obese does not guarantee that a person has or will have heart disease, but it does increase the risk, especially at the higher ranges of obesity. With obesity, risks for high blood pressure, elevated levels of triglycerides and cholesterol (especially low-density lipoprotein [LDL] and very-low-density lipoprotein [VLDL]), diabetes, and joint dysfunction all increase. The risks for heart attacks and strokes also increase with greater obesity; for African American women, this is a particularly ominous situation. Since heart disease affects women more severely in general and Black women are the most overweight, the risk factors for heart disease in all forms get amplified. Blacks are 90 percent more likely than Whites to die of a stroke. When you consider these factors together, it in part explains some of the reasons why Black women are the only group of Americans for whom heart disease statistics significantly worsened over the last 10 years.

If we look at the statistics for Black men, they are different as a group. They are not as overweight as Black women are. While Black men have a slightly higher incidence of death from coronary heart disease compared to White men,[1] Black women have a much higher in-cidence of coronary heart disease than do White women.

Much of the American population is overweight or obese; this issue is not unique to Black women. As a nation, we are collectively fatter now than we have ever been in the past, and this includes our young children and teenagers.

African American children receive mixed messages about weight and weight control. As we mentioned earlier, some girls are encouraged to gain weight. At the same time, other African American children, who are fat, are sometimes harassed for being fat by their family and their childhood peers, despite the widespread acceptance of obesity in the Black community. This creates a no-win situation. It is hard for a child (or adult) to handle being criticized by family and friends for ample body size and then be offered the very food items that can cause obesity by these same family members and friends. The food items asso-ciated with love, comfort, and acceptance are usually the starches and sugars (carbohydrates) that cause insulin levels to rocket in the blood-stream. Since insulin is the body's premier fat-building and fat storage hormone, all those excess carbohydrates just get turned into fat. This is especially pronounced in anyone whose metabolism is slowed or who has diabetes. These mixed messages about body size, food, emotional support, love, and peer or family approval of physical appearance can really send self-worth into a tailspin.

Some people are not greatly influenced by the opinions of others, while others are much more sensitive to these usually unsolicited opinions, criticisms, and feedback. The emotional dynamics at play can lead to a real challenge for an obese African American, and she or he may feel in part that if they lose the excess weight, they are somehow losing a part of their cultural or family identity, which may jeopardize self-esteem. This possible sense of loss can greatly interfere with other-wise constructive efforts to maintain weight at a healthful level.

People I have interviewed about what it is like to be fat consis-tently tell me that they feel they are told in lots of ways that it will take a miracle for them to get the weight off and keep it off. Part of the root of the issue lies in how they are treated by family and friends. Being made the butt of jokes hurts. My patients also report being told

"I love you" with food. This often happens during times of celebration and holidays, when loved ones might make special treats like pies for the fat person (usually high in fat, sugar, and salt), and then comment shortly after the meal about how fat that person is. This is a classic mixed message and helps keep the fat person trapped in the cycle of believing that weight loss involves miracles and that they are helpless—doomed by either the number or the size of the fat cells they have. It would be far more useful to go for a walk with your overweight loved one, encouraging and supporting their health-affirming choices and providing resources and accurate information that he or she can use to learn about the elements of sustained weight loss.

Also, it is important to recognize that just because someone is fat, it does not mean that they want to do something about it. We do not have to agree—and in many cases, we won't—with someone else's choices about their behavior or their health. For people who are chronically fat, the possibility of weight loss may look quite hopeless. These folks have been lied to, misled, picked on, humiliated, and generally been made to feel that being fat is a fault. It is a very personal thing to repeatedly experience scorn and rejection for such a fundamental aspect of life as how one appears to others in the world.

For African American women to be so overrepresented in the overweight or obese category is bad news for our heart health. Women's issues of poor or distorted body image and eating disorders are often lost in the ongoing discussion of weight in the United States, the country with the biggest advertising budget on the planet for snacks and fast food, cosmetics, high fashion, and quick weight-loss plans. Please know that my point of view on obesity and being overweight is rooted in a quest to inform women about good health and not part of a narrow image of how society thinks women of any race or ethnicity should look.

What's the difference between being overweight and being obese? More than just words. Overweight is medically defined as weighing up to 20 percent more than normal for your height and bony frame. Heavily muscled people do not fit this definition, as muscle weighs 1.2 times as much as fat, and increased muscle tissue burns fat even when a person is at rest. Thus, a heavily muscled woman may weigh more but have smaller measurements overall. If you have a smaller than average bony frame, your ideal weight range is different from that of someone who is the same height but has a larger than average bony frame. This relative measurement is more accurate and takes into account the variations between people of different body builds.

Obesity is medically defined as weighing 20 percent or more above the weight considered normal for your height and bony frame. There are different levels of obesity. Obesity may be classified as mild (20–40 percent overweight), moderate (41–100 percent overweight), and severe (more than 100 percent overweight). Most women who are obese are in the range of either mild or moderate obesity.

When there is too much weight for your height and bony frame, you are at greater risk for heart disease. If no actions are taken to remove the extra weight, the heart disease will become more severe. The cause(s) for the obesity must be identified and dealt with or the problem will remain. As anyone who has participated in a fad diet, crash dieting, or other forms of metabolic manipulation will tell you, those approaches do not work. There are no miracle cures for being overweight or obese. It is a shame that people continue to be misled about what these diets really offer. Good money and energy get thrown away when people pursue plans that are incapable of producing the result of gradual and sustained weight loss.

Be honest about your real weight. If your weight is fine, that's great. If you do have a weight problem, face it for what it is. You cannot change or address a problem you do not admit you have. Don't allow yourself to be fooled by myths that are common among Black women, such as "my weight is OK, I just have a big frame." The fact that Blacks typically do have a denser (therefore heavier) bony frame means to some women that all extra weight is due to bone density. Not true. Be honest with yourself about your real bony frame and its contribution to your weight. It is true that a larger bony frame hides more weight from view than a smaller frame would, but carrying around excessive weight may cheat you of the health you deserve. It can cut the life you live short and compromise the quality of life you enjoy by curtailing more strenuous activities like hiking, running, or skating. Similarly, obsession with thinness is also misguided. Like most things in life, balance is the key. Strive for your ideal weight with a range on either side of 5 percent, give or take a little. This will avoid the numerous complications associated with obesity. If you are very well muscled, your ideal weight range on either side may vary by 10 percent or so.

In my opinion, the situation for Black women and heart disease is very hopeful, as nothing about the statistics suggests these current problems with heart disease have to be permanent. Each element is treatable and correctable in its own right. Whether the symptoms are high blood pressure, diabetes, being overweight, obesity, poor eating habits, lack of exercise, or anything else—with the right help and a willingness to change, Black women can get their desired results.

Communication Is Key

We Need to Ask Questions about Our Health—I think people have to take responsibility for their own health. The more they know about their choices, the more likely it is that they will make a choice based on the results they are after and take the consequences of their decisions into account. When people are ignorant about their health, they are at the mercy of others. If a health care provider makes an error, the patient is the one who has to live with the consequences of the error. Doctors are human, and mistakes are made despite the best of intentions. Finger pointing is not helpful at that juncture, and I have seen and heard of more harm inflicted through a person's ignorance about health and medicine than from any other cause. When it comes to the topics of health and medicine, what you do not know *can* kill you.

It seems to me that the language of medicine puts people off. When our doctors use words we do not understand, we may feel intimidated or inadequate, and we might not ask them to use language we can more easily understand. Anytime someone uses language we do not understand—when they use words that are not common in our normal everyday conversation—they have power over us. This, in part, explains some of the lingering mistrust and confusion many people feel toward professionals that use big or unusual words, including doctors. People are afraid that their ignorance will cost them something precious, and at the same time they are afraid to reveal their ignorance for fear the professional will somehow think less of them as a person.

Racism and sexism contribute on many different levels to the African American's hesitance to ask questions in the patient–health care provider relationship. Many health care providers are White and male. As a doctor, I have heard both my Black female and male patients explain that their reluctance to ask health-related questions of their White doctors and nurses—even though they really wanted answers—was because they feared playing out stereotypes about intelligence and educational level. While this is not a big deal for all African Americans, it definitely is a factor for some. This is one less obvious factor that influences overall health care and how some decisions are made about health.

If numerous Black people withhold their questions about health and as a result get less than complete care, of course that will be reflected in discouraging health statistics. If White health care providers are racist, sexist, or simply insensitive, then it is not likely that they will work at making sure their patients are comfortable enough to ask whatever is on their minds. It is possible that their communication with their White or male patients or with patients with whom they have more in common (at least on the surface) will be adequate. The simple fact that a patient reminds them of their mom, brother, cousin, or niece can influence how they treat the patient, for better or worse. These kinds of dynamics are part of the reason why health-oriented attempts at community outreach are sometimes unsuccessful in predominantly African American communities. Some of these issues in the Black community may be attributable more to economic class than necessarily to race, ethnicity, or gender. Because skin color is a more obvious trait to some extent than economic status, it is easy to make assumptions based on skin color that may have nothing to do with the situation at all.

While I am not recommending that you turn into a control freak, I do recommend that you take reasonable precautions and make the effort to know and understand what is being done on behalf of your health. The same recommendation applies to your financial wealth. It is in your own best interests to find out what's going on and to know all your options. Professionals of all types are there to serve you and your best interests, not other agendas or conflicts of interest. My recommendation applies equally whether the health care you seek is conventional, natural, alternative, complementary, or goes by any other name.

Mistrust from Past Events—I have noticed that people from my grandparents' generation did not go to the doctor unless they felt it was absolutely necessary. My grandparents lived in the northeastern United States and had some access to medical doctors and osteopathic physicians. The northeastern United States did not have the formal expression of Jim Crow laws as rigidly enforced as they were in the South. Even so, there was a general feeling of mistrust concerning doctors. It was a common saying among the older African American members of my community that the folks who stayed away from the doctor's office lived longer. This saying represented a group perception that I have also heard expressed by my elderly White patients, especially if they were raised in the South. I think that some of what is being expressed is part of a generation-gap phenomenon, in which people who lived through the great economic depression of the 1930s feel less need to depend on medical professionals for their basic health needs. Some of this may be because in the earlier part of the 1900s, the medical profession's techniques and tools of the trade were not yet well refined. It may also reflect a lack of access to care, either due to inability to pay for the doctor's service or simply not being made to feel welcome in the doctor's office because of race or perceived economic status. Some residual behavioral compensation lingers today; some people go out of their way to dress very nicely when going to the doctor's office, even though they are quite ill and not feeling well at all.

Issues of access to the medical profession were also affected by whether there were enough doctors in a neighborhood to serve the needs of the community. The issue of access to medical care continues today; doctors were, and still are, typically found in greater numbers in more affluent neighborhoods and in more densely populated areas. Rural, sparsely populated, or poor areas often have significantly fewer medical providers than are needed. I am told by a colleague who grew up in the South that in that region, doctors were not used by poor people of any race because of cost and accessibility. Blacks also did not go to the doctor because of racism, as most of the White doctors would refuse to see non-White patients, especially Blacks. Blacks and poor Whites used herbalists, midwives, and family members for their health needs as much as possible. This social and economic dynamic did not help to build a bond of trust between these members of the community and the doctors who were supposed to serve them.

Sadly, there are added reasons for mistrust. Two particularly infamous episodes stand out in the history of medicine as it applies to African Americans.

One is the infamous Tuskegee, Alabama, study conducted over several decades. Five hundred ninety-nine Black men were the subjects of an experiment conducted without their permission or knowledge. The purpose of the experiment was to learn what the long-term effects of syphilis were if the disease was left untreated. These men were selected to be in this experiment, but no one asked them if they wanted to partici-pate. No one told them that an experiment was being conducted. The men thought they were receiving treatment over the decades. Obviously, they were lied to—treatment was deliberately withheld. This shows what can happen when you go into a situation where the balance of power is not in your hands. You are in the position of having to trust others, and your own ignorance about what is going on prevents you from keeping the people you are trusting honest and accountable. This sad episode of exploitation demonstrates the possible misuse of science and scientific methods to serve racist and other less than noble agendas.

The second episode concerns the use of Black slave women as unwil-ling models for testing and experimentation in the process of developing instruments that are now used as part of modern gynecological practice. A White Southern medical doctor used the bodies of Black slave women to develop the instruments. These women were not asked for their per-mission to serve as gynecological models; they were forced to comply. Perhaps mistrust of doctors can in part be attributed to a group memory of this and other undocumented abuse. Many women are very uncomfort-able with gynecological examinations, in part because of emotional dis-comfort or pain. I think that the way the exam is often conducted likely brings up feelings of extreme vulnerability. Such a physical examination can sometimes be the gateway to feelings, memories, and emotions of abuse or being forced to do something against one's will, such as rape or incest. While this is not every woman's experience (thank goodness!), for some women it can be a such a powerful trigger that they avoid any kind of physical examination that could possibly include their pelvic area, groin, or genitalia. If this is an issue for you, please deal with it in whatever way works for you so that you no longer allow it to prevent you from getting qualified, respectful medical help. Don't allow feelings based in the past (yours or your ancestors) to keep you from getting the help you need today with your health.

Abuses and harmful, hurtful interactions such as these remained fresh in Black folks' minds, and, combined with lack of access to doctors, racism, and poverty, it all adds up to not always trusting medical professionals the way other groups of Americans did or do. I believe that the legacy of slavery, racism, sexism, and poverty unfortunately continues to play out in the lives of African Americans and the daily choices we make concerning our health and how we take care of ourselves, or neglect to do so. If you don't get the message from somewhere that you really are worth something, that you really do count, then it might be pretty tough to come to that conclusion on your own.

African American women have a higher frequency of cancers of the breast, uterus, and ovaries. I have often wondered if it is simply that we neglect to take appropriate care of our health. Do we not know what to do? Do we not know early warning signs of trouble? Or is it that we do not get thorough yearly physical exams and therefore miss out on the screening opportunity these annual checkups represent? Please seek out qualified help, as today we have access to the most resources we have ever had in pursuit of health. Our ancestors did not have these options; we do.

Mental, Emotional, and Spiritual Factors

In the next sections, I offer my perspectives about some less tangible aspects of African American women's heart health today. I believe that the aftermath and consequences of slavery remain unhealed in our collective psyche. I also believe that this ongoing spiritual wound continues to affect our lives, and it is showing up in our poor heart health and heart disease. We must address any lingering remnants of distress, rage, resentment, fear, terror, and anything else that may feel unresolved, or we risk passing these things on unconsciously to our children.

Note: Some of the next sections on slavery and its aftereffects are graphic.

If you are easily offended, or do not wish to consider the details, skip ahead to the sections toward the end of the chapter, where there is a ritual for closure concerning slavery.

The Trauma of Slavery —It really is not much wonder that Black women are the only group for which the statistics on heart disease have worsened over the last 10 years. When you step back and consider that the Black women who were slaves in the United States never had an opportunity to really heal from the ongoing heartbreak of the extreme harshness of their lives, it seems inevitable that the heart would be susceptible to illness. By today's standards, the continual hardships and cruelty our foremothers and forefathers endured defy any sense of what we consider to be plain human decency. The meanness and evils that the slave women and men were subjected to in their daily lives were extreme.

The Middle Passage—Slavery existed in the New World for over four hundred years—twenty generations. That is, there was slavery in the Americas before Europeans began importing African as slaves. The strain on the African people who survived that trip across the Atlantic Ocean was tremendous. This forced journey of terror is now referred to as the "Middle Passage." The harrowing journey, which lasted six weeks or more, was completed without adequate food or water, without opportunity for personal hygiene or for defecating in a sanitary manner. Many of the Africans captured for the slave trade died during the Middle Passage because of dehydration, hunger, terror, and the squalor on the transport ships. Those who survived did not expect that opportunity was awaiting them when they arrived on foreign soil.

Some people theorize that those who survived the Middle Passage, the strong ones, may have had an unusual ability to retain salt in their blood. This trait would help them stay hydrated enough to survive the ordeal of too little water for too many people on board the slave ships. This same ability to retain salt, and therefore water, which may have helped them survive the Middle Passage, would leave these people more vulnerable to the water-retaining effects of salt in the bloodstream—and, therefore, specifically leave them vulnerable to the possible development of hypertension (high blood pressure). It might in part explain why

African Americans as a group seem much more prone to high blood pressure than other groups in the United States and Africans in Africa, our predominant genetic family members. Some studies have shown that our physiological use of sodium is different than that of Whites.[2] African Americans have been shown to be deficient in blood levels of potassium and calcium, specific minerals that help to decrease the blood-pressure-raising effects of sodium in those who are susceptible to hypertension.[3]

Physical and Sexual Abuse—Consider the relentless heartbreak of Black slave women. Think for a moment about their experience of having their children repeatedly stolen from them and sold. The women were raped over and over again by slave owners, plantation owners, plantation overseers, and anyone else who had power over them and was in a position to get away with this assault. These women had no control over keeping lovers, husbands, and children by their side as they too were sold away, murdered, or beaten senseless. They wondered when the pain would end, hoping against hope that one day something that was fair or at least better than their current situation would actually happen in their lives. They dared to dream of a day when they, their sweethearts, and their children would be truly free. This harsh history could magnify the effects of all of the risk factors for heart disease and multiply the impact of any single factor to ensure that heart disease would have a huge, disproportionate impact in this particular community of the world's women.

The women felt rage over being taken sexually without their consent or permission; fury at being forced to do things that they did not want to do with people they probably hated; outrage at the unfairness of the situations; and despair over whether things would ever be better or different. Some slaves were overcome with despair, so much so that they committed suicide rather than continue on in slavery. Some showed defiance—soon-to-be slaves recently captured in western Africa sometimes jumped overboard from slave ships rather than finish the journey to the "New World," where they would become slaves in an unknown land with unknown people, foods, languages, and weather.

Today uterine fibroids, cancers of the breasts, uterus, and ovaries affect African American women more frequently than other groups of women. I think that some of the reason for the increased frequency of these particular diseases lies in the unhealed (and perhaps unrecognized) energetic memory, the imprint of the sexual trauma our slave ancestors endured.

Forced Separation—Black slave women had their children stolen from them and sold off to other plantations. The mothers had no say at all in this. Put yourself in the place of one of these women, and imagine how this feels; really feel it and just sit with it for a while. Allow the reality of this predicament to soak in. Consider that if she protested the sale of her children in any way, she risked murder, rape, sodomy, lynching, severe beatings, torture, starvation, and other punishments for simply trying to keep her children by her side.

Many parents—especially mothers—experience a strong sense of loss when their children go off to school, leave for college, or get married. We can only imagine the incredible sorrow, grief, and heartbreak our ancestors felt as they watched their children being sold off, beaten, murdered, or otherwise mistreated according to the whims of the slave owners.

What was it like for these women to watch as their children were taken away? What was the anguish these Black slave women felt as they saw their children repeatedly harmed in various ways? They saw their lovers and husbands taken away. They saw the men beaten, sold off, or murdered before their very eyes. What was it like for these women as they dealt with how they felt about being beaten themselves, raped, and abused over and over again? They saw their sisters, mothers, aunts, and cousins abused and murdered. How did these Black women compensate for the tremendous and ongoing losses they experienced? Did their hearts routinely skip beats as a response to the ongoing terror that filled their lives?

Slavery represents a blight across all the realms of human experience—physical, mental, emotional, and spiritual. It really was a kind of social and economic cancer, choking the life out of otherwise healthy people. It was harmful to both the African slaves and to the Whites who owned them.

I think the overall consequence is that heart health was negatively affected across the board. A bomb called slavery set off a whole series of reactions and compensations: some physical, others spiritual, mental, and emotional. From what we know today about body language and behavior, when someone looks down, they experience a feeling of being down, depressed, or pessimistic; when they look up, they feel more positive and optimistic. Slaves didn't get to look their owners in the eyes. Having their heads held high and shoulders back wasn't welcome; it was not part of the psychology of keeping a group of people under control. Early on, slave parents taught their children to keep their eyes down to help them survive the indoctrination and increase the odds of their survival to adulthood. These children learned it well and passed it on to the next generation.

Yet, even in the face of the horrors of slavery, the spiritual heart is a wondrous thing to behold. It has infinite capacity to recover, given reasonable opportunity to do so. My grandparents would say that "time heals all wounds." How true this is. Yet I have observed that when the spiritual impact of a wrong is big enough, the spiritual heart may need more than time to heal. The compensations that people develop after they've been repeatedly wronged or survived a major trauma can develop psychological and spiritual roots of their own. For example, a person who has repeatedly experienced betrayal may decide that trusting anyone is not safe, and she will keep herself from trusting others for fear that they will hurt her. It takes a lot of energy to build and maintain those personal walls. To keep from building those walls, this person would have to be willing to trust people anyway, recognizing that she remains vulnerable and that she can protect herself better next time or recover as need be. She must see that there is nothing so big that she cannot heal and recover from it. If all of the roots of the compensations are not destroyed, then they can create all sorts of gummy little associations that leave people with less of a life than they otherwise would have created and enjoyed.

To really recover fully from major upset, the spiritual heart needs time and effective tools like laughter, crying, rest, and the opportunity to heal. I think that the slaves rarely, if ever, had the needed circumstances to really heal from their experience of slavery. I believe that the genetic and emotional consequences of this lack of healing for the spiritual heart are part of what was passed on to us from our slave ancestors. It is not their fault in any way, shape, or form; these people were truly doing the best they could with what they had. While we know they had little in the way of physical possessions, it's past time that we acknowledged that the African slaves had a tremendous ability to survive a situation that was not set up for their well-being at all. Their "possessions" were more of a spiritual and mental nature, and we have inherited them through all of our generations.

The Culmination of Emotional Abuse—When someone is upset or fearful, they may feel some of their distress in the area of their stomach; if they are frightened, they may shake and tremble. There are lots of ways that our feelings and emotions are expressed physically, even though that is not the realm from which they originated.

Today we know that people register and store memories of emotional trauma in their physical bodies. With this ability then, it is likely that stored memories of trauma can be passed on just as other family traits are passed on to the next generation, either because of genetic influences and expression or through family and other social habits.

Spiritual anxieties, knots, and kinks in one's soul, can show up as chronic illness that is poorly defined, even to the person whose health has been compromised. In the field of mind-body medicine, much research is under way to help explain and quantify these processes, as they are powerful and often silent, even to the people stuffing their feelings down. Since we don't live in test tubes, it can be hard to do this kind of research and get it published; it doesn't fit neatly into the model of "control" groups (unaffected reference groups) for part of the experiment. This means that for future generations, issues of self-esteem are not addressed. The work concerning the emotional heart still needs to be done. The spiritual heart still needs to be fed and nurtured. Being optimistic and having hope for your future includes taking the actions that help ensure that your future is a healthy one and realizing that fundamentally you deserve to be happy, healthy, and feel whole. This may explain in part why African Americans as a group still do not take full advantage of the health resources they have at their disposal today. Some of us are acting as if it is still illegal for us to go to the doctor, or to cry and not have it all together all the time, or to plan for our future. At the heart of things, it seems that we don't think we have a future or deserve to treat ourselves really well with the things that matter. Instead, we try to cover our psychic wounds with shiny baubles and an "I'm strong, I can take anything" attitude. Inappropriate expression of strength is a trap. In this context, it is really bravado, and it prevents the full expression of normal emotions, feelings, and spirituality.

Heartbreak: A Universal Theme in the Human Experience—Most languages of the world have words that express the sentiment of "heartbreak." When a theme is universal, you know that it is an important aspect of being human. It is something we all have in common as people on our planet, Earth.

What role did the inevitable emotional and spiritual knots that developed play in how slave women raised their children? How did they give their children the best chances for survival in the slave world and at the same time keep the fires of freedom burning so that their children would always know that a better life was possible and that this better life was for them? I believe there was an emphasis on discipline and strict enforcement of rules so that the children would be under control at an early age. Slave children did not get to be as expressive as children normally are; whining, arguing with authority figures, and defying the rules were not tolerated. Breaking these rules meant risking severe punishment.

The heartbreak the slaves endured, then, was not just the heartbreak of loss and personal degradation. It was also the heartbreak of lost childhood and innocence. To survive, slaves always had to be defensive and on guard. They did not have the freedom to be open, to express who they really were. Perhaps their hearts broke, both literally and figuratively, with the weight of all they had to bear, all they had to hold in, and all they could not share.

The Physical Consequences of Slavery

The Effects of Vitamin Deficiency on Our Ancestors —We know from historical analysis that most slaves had a diet deficient in basic nutrients and that they did not live as long as their owners. The incidence of diseases like pellagra (caused by deficiency of thiamine, or vitamin B_1) and beriberi (caused by deficiency of niacin, or vitamin B_3) were much higher among slaves than the rest of the population. Medical care, such as it was in

those days, was withheld from slaves unless they were thought to be particularly valuable property—so slaves had to figure out their own health
solutions. Given their poor living conditions, slaves were more exposed
to the elements and more likely to die from infectious diseases. The slaves
who survived the brutality were really strong in many ways. I think the
lack of opportunity to heal and fully recover from the trauma of being a
slave meant that through nurture and physiology, they passed on
whatever was possible to pass on.

Living with Sustained Stress—With the benefit of today's science, we know
that the heart is greatly affected by feelings of grief, rage, and stress.
Slaves had all these feelings in abundance and very limited outlets for the
safe expression of these powerful emotions. Much like the slaves, Black
women today often feel powerless to express their true feelings—as the
cork gets stuffed ever tighter in the emotional bottle, blood pressure rises
higher and higher. Even intraocular (within the eyes) pressure rises when
tears and emotional upsets are stored instead of released. Stuffing down
feelings and appearing strong at all costs has very real consequences for
our health.

The chemicals produced by the body when we are under stress (such
as adrenaline) allow us to perform miracles when needed. You've heard
about small women lifting cars off of their children or people fleeing at
great speeds when chased by wild animals. Some of these stories are true.
However, these very same chemicals do great damage to the heart when
they run through our blood for no particular purpose or for no specific
call to action. In unrelieved stress situations, these chemicals damage the
heart tissue and blood vessels by weakening the lining of the blood
vessels. These weakened places in blood vessel linings then become the
sites where fatty deposits can accumulate.

Some hurts heal faster than others do, whether the hurts are
physical, mental, emotional, or spiritual in nature. It seems to me that
Black slave women and men had to make hard choices on a constant
basis about how they would deal with their harsh, extreme situation.
When did the slaves have the opportunity to wail for their losses, their
rage, their frustration and disappointments? Who cried for these
people? Did these women and men ever get to weep? Even today, men

in general are still discouraged from crying or expressing any emotions that might be perceived as weakness by others. This keeps men in a narrow little box that limits the emotions society permits them to express. For women, emotional expression is OK, but in the Black community, Black women may be pressured to appear strong at all costs for fear of making others uncomfortable. Or perhaps the emphasis on strength echoes a time when it was not safe or practical to show the world anything other than strength.

Surviving slavery required all sorts of compensations. If slaves were angry with their owner, they could not show that anger; if they did, they were punished severely, killed, or sold to another plantation. Instead, most of the time, these feelings of anger or rage were kept inside. Research shows that when people keep anger bottled up inside—especially if they say they do not feel stressed by a situation that most people would say causes them to feel stress—they tend to develop high blood pressure.[4] With today's science, we can directly link the suppression of certain feelings to the development of disease, in particular those that affect the heart and cardiovascular system. Anger turned inward is known to lead to depression, liver disorders, hypertension, heart attacks, heartburn, indigestion, and other diseases and ailments. The powerful feelings the slave women had to keep bottled up in an attempt to survive extreme situations must have had some impact on their health and the health of future generations.

Toni Morrison paints a horrifying and all-too-plausible scene in her novel and screenplay *Beloved,* in which the lead character, Sethe, murders her own child rather than see the child captured and returned to the world of slavery. The scene is a reminder that the slaves experienced terror in many ways. Fleeing in the night on foot to escape all that went with the slave world, fearing barking hound dogs, and smelling and hearing gunfire behind them as they ran away, was not uncommon. The intensity of these feelings must have been tremendous.

It is hard for us to imagine what these brave people must have endured. They must have tapped some deep reservoir from which they drew the courage and stamina required to survive the slave experience. It is a testimony to the power of these Black women's and men's spirits that they kept hope alive and did not give up. Many of them took every opportunity possible to run away and escape slavery themselves or at the very least help their children get safely to freedom.

In times of unprocessed grief, the heart feels heavy to its owner, the blood circulation becomes sluggish, and the body's energy begins to stagnate. Carried forward in time, the grief, rage, and stress multiply. The effect each one has can create a time bomb of impending heart disease. The body and mind are definitely connected and interact all the time. It is not possible or practical to separate the body from the mind, nor our spirit from either.

The Effects of Slavery on Our Well-Being Today

The effects of slavery are far-reaching—physically, emotionally, and spiritually. Let's take a closer look at how the legacy of slavery touches us today.

Putting Our Hearts on the Line

We just don't want to take the chance of putting our hearts on the line one more time, only to feel like we've been rejected again and made to feel bad for who we are and what we look like. Historically, we have been the target of jokes, caricatures, abuse, and violence—all of which was done simply because we're Black. In my opinion, our ancestors' experience of slavery as well as continuing racism has left a residual heartache—a sickness imprint—on the hearts of all African Americans. Under certain conditions, that imprint can lead to illness and make that illness more severe and more deadly than it otherwise would be if we didn't share this difficult collective history.

What are the consequences we face for carrying over these internalized emotions and behavioral compensations as part of the legacy of slavery? What are the consequences for our current rates of heart disease? How many of us as African American women and men in today's world have fully healed or completely recovered from the mental, emotional, and spiritual damage left by slavery? The people who were sold into slavery are physically dead now. Does that mean that slavery and everything to do with it is dead now too? Does it mean there are no lingering consequences, or does the impact of that brutal episode of dehumanization live on? I think that it does live on and that it explains the current reality that Black women die earlier of heart disease and experience more severe forms of heart disease than other groups of people.

The imprint left by slavery on the emotional and spiritual heart of the descendents of slaves continues to this day. Although much has changed since those times—we can now legally vote, own property, read, write, and participate fully in what this country has to offer—we still don't treat ourselves as well as we should. I don't mean spending money on fancy clothes or buying expensive trinkets. I am talking about putting our health and personal needs first. I think we sometimes scale back our own ambitions because we don't want to face further disappointments. I think sometimes as parents we caution our children to not expect too much from life or other people because we don't want them to be disappointed. We've been conditioned to think this way. It's a tactic we use to keep our children relatively safe and out of trouble, because historically it was not safe for us to call attention to ourselves or our children. Parents who use this approach are probably trying to soften the sting of racism or sexism.

Black Women and Rage

Have you ever felt rage that was out of proportion to the event that prompted it? Have you felt fury so intense that you knew you could kill anyone who got in your way just because it would be a release from this emotional hurricane? Have you ever had an experience you knew was not completely your own—you felt as if it belonged to someone else from another time and space?

Over the years, many African American women have shared with me their experiences with rage. At times they were so swept up in this inner fury that they responded by turning the rage outward, striking out at anything and everything, not caring (in the moment) about the consequences. When I listen to these experiences and remember my own episodes of rage, I see a common thread: we all know that the intensity of our response may not be entirely based in the present. Despite this semblance of objectivity, we are at least partially consumed by the raging fire and do or say things we later regret. Often we had no conscious idea we felt this rage, but obviously it was inside us somewhere, waiting to come out. I wonder if some of the rage that is out of proportion to present circumstances remains as rage our slave ancestors never got to express and process due to the harsh reality of their lives. Something to think about, isn't it?

Where Are We Today?

Is it possible that the horror of slavery was recorded genetically and transmitted to future generations of African Americans? Could it be that any major hurt, if it is not healed completely in our lifetime, could be passed on either genetically or via our family and cultural behavior patterns?

Is there a resonance phenomenon other than genetics that passes on both the good and the bad that our ancestors have to share with us all? In homeopathy, this idea is expressed in the concept of miasms. Esoteric studies express the idea of the ether, a morphogenetic (structural development) field that exists across time and space and represents a grid where we experience present time reality intermingled with the unresolved elements of our individual and collective pasts. The proposed existence of such things implies that until we individually and collectively heal from the legacy of slavery, anything that is not resolved will continue to play itself out forward in time. If, in an invisible way, the past is determining the future, then it is critical to clean up anything from the past that could jeopardize the future.

Issues of rage, trust, betrayal, loyalty, courage, compassion, fear, terror, and hope were intertwined for Black slave women, creating a kind of emotional cloth that describes their struggle to survive each day. The richness and depth of a beautiful, traditional fabric such as *kente* cloth (which is still woven and produced in Africa) speaks to our cultural capability to deal with complexity and weave it into the ordinary elements of life, creating a cloth that symbolizes wholeness that is both beautiful and functional.

There is a premium on fully healing any and all old and current hurts associated with slavery. Our current and future health status may depend on our collective and individual ability to clean up any residual mess from the days of slavery. Many people would rather not look at this period of American history, and that is unfortunate. Ignoring it won't make it go away, so we might as well step up to what needs to happen for some real healing to take place. Let's all move on with our lives.

Embracing the Past to Reclaim the Future: A Healing Response

The past and how we feel about it can only chain us if we let it. It is far better to burst free of the mental and spiritual shackles than to allow any leftover effects of the slave experience to have a negative effect on our lives today or in the future. Slavery legally ended in 1865. Jim Crow laws remained in effect until the 1970s. We have arrived at a new century and a new millennium. It is time to cast off the things that no longer serve us and only keep those things that help us live wonderful lives—things that allow us to be the very best we can be. We can now read, write, have careers, receive equal pay, make use of the courts of law, get insurance policies, own real estate, and do all the other things that White Americans were never excluded from by law based on the color of their skin. Granted, the centuries of slavery represent lost income and the wealth that could have been inherited had our ancestors had the opportunity to accumulate financial wealth, but it is time to move on.

I for one am grateful to my African ancestors for their refusal to settle for anything less than full participation in American society. I realize that I am the recipient of the fruits of their unshakable faith. I also appreciate the efforts of all people who were allies in the fight to make things right, the non-Blacks who supported progress in whatever way they could. Thank you to everyone.

But sisters, it is time to wail. Really feel all that bottled-up grief, rage, anger, disappointment, shock, and everything else that got all jumbled up in slavery. These powerful feelings have been held inside for centuries. It's time to release them and leave room for the things we enjoy and that help us to thrive. There is some seriously stuck *qi* (pronounced "chee") around this issue. It is time to move all the clogged, congested energy on its way.

Our ancestral moms and grandmoms couldn't go where they needed to go emotionally to complete their own healing because their situation was so extreme, so very harsh. Their worries for the future of our collective safety and actual existence kept them from wailing out loud, lashing out, crying, and doing all the things folks do to heal from the intensity of these hurts. We get to do this work.

Know that as you work through your own grief about what happened during slavery, you are being watched and loved by your ancestors. They are all around us. We are not alone in this or anything else. Our ancestors cheer us on every time we do anything that allows us as individuals and as a group to heal our past. These same spirits cheer whenever we take the steps needed to live a full and rewarding life.

Dealing with this mess is a must. Just as a thorough housecleaning does wonders for the appearance of our homes and how we feel about our homes, an emotional cleanse is needed to purge forever any residual junk left from our ancestors' slave experience. Take the good and eliminate the rest.

What could possibly be good about this, you ask? The first thing that comes to mind is the extraordinary strength and grace our ancestors maintained to bear this oppression and live through it.

That any person of African ancestry in the United States could ever doubt their personal power is ridiculous. There is no reason to think "I can't do/be/have _____ ." No reason whatsoever. Our ancestors worked so very hard for our freedom. Some slaves, against formidable obstacles, actually saved up enough money to buy their own freedom and the freedom of their spouse, children, and other family members. Historical statistics show that approximately one in nine slaves bought their own freedom and/or purchased freedom for loved ones.

Slaves struggled to get the opportunity to read and write, to vote, and to participate as full and equal members in the larger American society. They stayed focused on their goals and kept on keepin' on until they got what they sought. So, we know we can do it too. There's a wealth of history that proves over and over the abundance of spirit of the people we come from. Tap into it where needed and make the best use of it. This is our heritage.

Once enough work has been done with the issues about the past, especially issues based in slavery and repercussions from slavery times, it is relatively easy to move forward in our lives and claim what we want for ourselves. Old disappointments and upsets become exactly that—old stuff. Goals become clearer and resources are put to good use. We create our own opportunities and use our heritage of practical flexibility and making something out of what appears to be nothing work for us instead of for someone else.

Now is the time, and we are the ones to make it happen.

Cleansing from the Legacy of Slavery: A Ritual for Closure

I offer the ritual at the end of this chapter as a place to begin in working through remaining issues from slavery. If you feel you have no lingering issues about slavery or associations to it, then perhaps you can use this ritual for closure around anything else bugging you, such as racism, sexism, or economic disparity.

It is important to acknowledge what has happened in the past—any past—and take what was good about it and transform anything that was bad into something good. Any of the events in our lives or our ancestors' lives only mean what we want them to mean, no more and no less. We get to choose the meaning, so let's assign useful meanings and associations to this legacy so we can all move on and experience the majesty that is possible in our lives today. You'll be amazed at how much energy can be reclaimed when you do a cleansing ritual, so let us continue the healing process.

Lay These Burdens Down

The heavy heart can be unburdened. Healing is possible. Healing means different things to different people. As long as you know what healing and health mean to you, you can establish and nourish the foundations of health, especially heart health. While our ancestral mothers who were slaves may not have had the opportunity to fully lay their burdens down, today it is truly different. Each of us gets to make that choice to heal, to let go of whatever does not serve us, and to keep what works well for us. There is no magic fix for heart problems. Rewards will come from regular efforts addressed to what has gone wrong when it comes to health, including heart health. Positive actions taken every day are what create a healthy heart.

Looking in the rearview mirror has its use when driving a car. So does looking forward through the windshield, watching where you are going on your path. Balance is the key.

Learn from the past. Savor the present. Create the future.

We get what we expect in life. It's time to expect more, and get it.

---

[1] American Heart Association, *1999 Heart and Stroke Statistical Update* (Dallas, Texas: American Heart Association, 1999), 10.

[2] Clarence E. Grim, et al., "Electrolyte and Volume Homeostasis in Blacks," in *Hypertension in Blacks: Epidemiology, Pathophysiology and Treatment*, ed. W. D. Hall et al. (Chicago: Year Book Medical Publishers, 1985), 115–6, 118, 123, 125, 128.

[3] Ibid., 122–4, 126.

[4] Derek W. Johnston. *Mind-Body Medicine: A Clinician's Guide to Psychoneuroimmunology*, ed. Alan Watkins (New York: Churchill Livingstone, 1997), 75–85.

Cleansing Ritual

*Create a quiet time and space where you can do this work undisturbed.
Consider inviting others whom you are close to and trust to do this work
with you.*

Items needed: plenty of paper to write on, pen or pencil, matches or
open grill, and a surface you can burn items on, one glass of pure
water, a bowl, and a dry towel.

1. Put aside about 10 pieces of paper or so to write on at the end of
   the ritual.
2. State what your intentions are in doing this ritual.
3. Say these words out loud.
4. Pour the pure water into a bowl.
5. Wash your hands and face with the pure water.
6. Dry off.
7. Write down all the bad things that you associate with slavery, especially as it relates to the lives of the Black slave women. Write
   until you can't write any more.
8. Take some deep, belly-lifting breaths and repeat step 7 until you
   are completely empty of anything else to write.
9. Now write down anything in your current life that is not the way
   you want it to be, especially if you think it could have roots in the
   legacy of slavery. Include any places where you hold yourself back,
   especially if you are not sure why you seem to get in your own way.
10. Rip up these pieces of paper; really shred them.
11. Pile up these pieces of paper.
12. Burn this pile of paper. Watch the flames as they consume the
    paper.
13. As the papers become embers, conjure up anything you wish to
    release that no longer serves you.

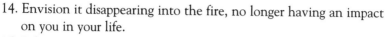

14. Envision it disappearing into the fire, no longer having an impact on you in your life.
15. Take some more deep, belly-expanding breaths.
16. Let the feelings wash over you, notice what you feel and think now.
17. Write down what you experienced: the feelings, thoughts, sounds, smells, sensations, whatever came through to you as you did this work.
18. Wash your hands and face with the pure water.
19. Dry off.

Congratulations on daring to go where few have gone before.
Repeat this ritual as necessary for your personal sense of completion.

Chapter 3
The Impact of Heart Disease on Black Women's Lives

The choices we make in our lives and the consequences of these choices often become much clearer to us when illustrated through an anecdote. I shared a personal story with you in the beginning of the book to give you a framework for the significance of this information. I hope that it pointed out how crucial it is to make use of what you know to take care of yourself before it is too late. Stories appear throughout this book as a way to help you really understand how our daily habits determine the level of health we enjoy. African tradition is rich in the history of the griot, the storyteller. My purpose here is to invoke the educational tools of this tradition in the stories I share here.

Sharon's Story

One day Sharon noticed that she really didn't feel well. This overall sense of feeling poorly had sort of sneaked up on her bit by bit over time. When friends and family asked her how she was, she always said, "I am just fine, thank you. And how are you?" If Sharon said that now, she'd be telling a lie. The one thing she did not feel was fine. It seemed lately that she couldn't put on enough antiperspirant. She was breaking out into a sweat easily, and she wasn't even going through "the change"; that happened years ago. What had started months ago as mild headaches had now become severe, and she swore at times it felt like her heart was beating so hard it was going to come out right through her chest. Simple activities like going up and down steps at home were major events lately, using up what little energy she had.

Sharon knew something wasn't right, but she wasn't quite sure what was wrong. Every time she thought about getting help for herself, she got distracted by some other "crisis" at work or at home. People at work counted on her to come through in the crunch since she was the one who could handle stress best. As deadlines approached, Sharon was the one who got things done and made it happen time and again.

"Steady as a rock," her coworkers said.

"She makes it look so easy. It hardly even looks like she's working," commented others.

"When you need a miracle, go to Sharon," said her manager.

With this kind of feedback on her job and her role of caretaker at home, Sharon didn't feel quite right about putting her needs first by taking time to exercise and eat healthy meals. After all, the people at work were counting on her. When she did take time to eat at work, she ate really fast, practically inhaling her food in just a few bites. Chew? Who had time to actually chew food? Swallowing it whole was a better way to describe the way she usually ate her food. For Sharon, it was fast food, snack food, or no food at all.

The situation at home was not much different. Viewed as the family crisis resource, she got calls for help all the time from her sister, brother, and her children. How could she say no? All of her family members depended on her. And yet she felt physically ill most of the time now, so bad that she was getting scared something serious might be wrong. Headaches, easy and profuse sweating, fatigue, and a pervasive sense of not feeling well were her constant companions.

Well, if something is wrong, Sharon thought, I'll just take a pill or two to fix the problem and it will go away. The day Sharon went to the doctor's office for the results of her physical exam and lab work was a day of personal revelation. She learned that not only did she have high blood pressure, she also had really high cholesterol and triglyceride levels, her fasting blood sugar was too high, she was well on her way to being obese, and if she didn't make major changes now, she was at serious risk for a heart attack, a stroke, diabetes, or a combination of these three.

Sharon was shocked. "How could this become so bad so fast? Did I just fall apart over night?" she asked.

"No," her doctor responded. "Sharon, these problems take time to develop. This didn't just happen to you out of the blue. And to change this situation, you must change how you live."

Sharon sighed and let the information sink in. Realizing that nothing good could come of ignoring her situation any longer, she decided it was time for a change. Sharon took the steps needed in her personal life and on the job to make her health her first priority. She had to put herself first or risk prolonged, serious illness—even death—if she neglected herself any further. Those steps involved changes in her eating habits, exercise patterns, and stress management. Sharon made priorities of creating time for relaxation and learning how to use the word "no."

Do you recognize yourself or someone you care about in Sharon's story? She genuinely felt that she couldn't "find the time" to exercise and eat well. Sharon didn't yet understand that she had to *make* the time to take care of herself by arranging her day around exercise and good meals, getting up earlier and going to sleep sooner, if needed, to support good health habits. Her current habit of putting her own needs last was causing her to lose ground on any reasonable hope of living long and living well as she got older. It also jeopardized her current level of health.

Sharon's perception of time is shared by many people with health habits similar to hers. She thought that to change her behaviors she needed to find time in an already overcrowded daily schedule. The internal shift she needed to make was to realize that there is no such thing as "finding time." Time is both a relative perception and an objective taskmaster. It is one of the few truly fair things in life. Everyone gets the same amount of time in a day. Time does not play favorites by giving some folks 25 hours in a day and cheat others with just 22.

For Sharon's health habits to change, she had to stop using "I don't have time" as reason number one for not taking better care of herself.

As I often say to my patients, if you tell yourself you don't have time to exercise, eat well, get enough rest, and take care of yourself, then what you are really telling yourself is that you do have time to be sick and feel bad. It really is a matter of priorities. Sometimes activities or obligations have to be juggled or dropped altogether to get your needs back on the schedule. I have worked with people with amazing schedules and life responsibilities, and they have all been able to make this shift about how they think about and make use of the time in their day. Such people make exercise the centerpiece of the daily schedule and prepare simple, nutritious meals in advance so that when they get busy during the day, they are eating food that is good for them and have already gotten their physical workout done. They feel better, have more energy, notice improved concentration, and have an upbeat attitude, all of which are key ingredients in leading a fulfilled life.

It's a Family Matter

It was a quiet summer day, a Sunday afternoon in the big city. The children and grandchildren were visiting. Lucy was 57 years old, at least 40 pounds overweight, smoked about a pack of cigarettes a day, and had not been to a doctor of any kind for many years. Lucy did not trust doctors and would not go for even so much as a checkup. Family members could not remember ever seeing her exercise except for extensive seasonal cleaning of her home for Easter, summertime, and Christmas. Except for time spent cooking, cleaning, and doing laundry, Lucy spent her days sitting down reading, doing puzzles, or watching TV.

Everyone had eaten breakfast earlier in their own homes before coming over, and they had just finished lunch together as a family. Breakfast, just like lunch, was full of foods with lots of fat, salt, sugar, and little fiber. Shortly after eating, Lucy began to behave oddly. She started to slur her words and not finish sentences when she was speaking. In fact, her usually lively conversation came to a complete halt. Over and over again, Lucy tried to put her house keys and other inappropriate objects resting on the kitchen table in her mouth, despite her daughters' repeated instructions to not do that. Her daughters were really puzzled. They could see clearly that something was wrong, but they didn't know what. Lucy's face began to droop on one side, drool came out of her mouth, and her eyes lost their shine. Her daughters called for emergency help and an ambulance.

The emergency medical technicians arrived quickly and got Lucy to the hospital. Family members followed the ambulance.

It was a stroke. After Lucy was admitted to the hospital, doctors told the family that it was not likely that she would regain much mental function or physical ability; the stroke was massive, causing severe brain damage. Lucy spent two weeks in a coma in the hospital's intensive care and cardiac care units before she died. Her husband, two daughters, two sons, and her grandchildren were devastated by her death. The loss was so sudden. The family had lost a precious member, one all of them dearly loved and looked up to.

After Lucy's death, the family grieved and gradually resumed their lives. Lucy's husband, Victor, had a mild heart attack two years after her death, followed by a silent stroke and massive heart attack that killed him in his sleep. Victor was a nonsmoker, drank about one alcoholic drink a day, did not exercise, and still ate the same way Lucy had (low fiber and high fat, salt, and sugar).

Again, the family grieved. At that point, all of the family members continued the lifestyle habits they had learned from their parents and grandparents. Everyone continued to eat a diet high in fat, sugar, and salt, and low in fiber, not knowing that this kind of nutrition had directly helped cause the early deaths of Lucy and Victor. The only family members that exercised regularly were a couple of athletic grandchildren; everyone else was sedentary, preferring to sit around rather than routinely participate in aerobic physical activity. The family emotional pattern stayed intact at that time; the response to stress was "Keep it to yourself." A frequently heard comment among the family was "We're strong; we can take it."

Any of this sound familiar? If so, consider that now so much more can be done to prevent heart disease and treat existing heart problems, but first, you must do your part. Go to the doctor's office; get your regular physical exams and blood tests; and keep up with eye exams, dental checkups, and fitness evaluations on a yearly basis. Investing in your health pays you back in quality of life and possibly quantity of life too. Days that are pain-free, full of energy and zest, are worth their weight in gold. If you doubt that, ask the opinion of anyone who no longer has their health.

Who's More Likely to Die of a Stroke?

Over the age of 65, the incidence of strokes is 19 percent higher for men than for women.[1] For persons 65 or younger, the difference is even higher. Yet the death rate from strokes is 20 percent higher for women (39.1 percent for men, 60.9 for percent women).[2] The upshot: Blacks have the same frequency as Whites for how often a stroke happens. The stunning difference is that Blacks are almost 90 percent more likely to *die* from a stroke than are Whites.

Stroke risk is driven by the factors of high blood pressure, smoking, and excessive alcohol consumption, and all of these factors affect Blacks more severely. We can also do something about these factors, provided that we are willing to make changes in our behavior patterns—the way we eat, exercise, handle stress, consume alcohol, and get rest.

Why is the death rate from strokes for Blacks so huge? Quality of life after the stroke is largely determined by how quickly help is sought and received after the person has the stroke. If they receive help in the first few critical hours, then the odds are favorable they will have a good recovery after they complete appropriate rehabilitation. If help was delayed for any reason, then the odds of a good recovery are not as favorable.

Help is most often delayed because the person having the stroke and the people around him or her do not know a stroke's warning signs. As we've already discussed, knowledge of these warning signs can be literally life saving. If you think you or someone you know is having a stroke, it's as important to get them to the emergency room right away as it is in the case of a heart attack. Similarly, denial that someone may be having a stroke or otherwise being slow to take action can waste precious time and keep the person from getting the help they need.

The Unholy Trio

Black Women and Obesity—Some Reasons Why

The degree to which we as African Americans are overweight in today's world is amazing, and it has to stop. Being chronically overweight or obese is collectively killing us, slow and sure. Recognize that this problem hasn't come on overnight and will not miraculously go away overnight either. Consistent, focused, rational efforts do pay off for most people when it comes to weight management.

Obesity is a multifaceted problem. It can be due to diabetic complications, thyroid problems, lack of exercise, genetic factors, poor quality foods, or simply eating too much. All of these are helped by natural treatment options including herbs, nutrition, counseling, and aerobic forms of exercise. Treatment options are explored in the following chapters.

Getting older is not the enemy, and time is not the enemy. Any perceived enemies or limitations can be transformed if you are willing to learn the lessons that either people or situations offer. Take the best meaning you can from it and move on. Dwelling on what you did not do, what you used to eat, or how much you smoked as a way to beat yourself up is not an effective way to make healthy changes last permanently.

African American women are the most overweight group in America today. The reasons are many. Traditional soul food preparations are high in fat and were developed during an era when we had significantly greater physical activity, working all day long on plantations. Today, foods typically eaten when celebrating with family and friends are high in fat, sugar, and salt. These foods get associated with good times early in childhood, and this makes it easy later in life to use food as a way to feel good, at least for the moment. In addition, levels of aerobic exercise and strength training are relatively low among Black women. Poor quality nutrition coupled with inadequate exercise contribute greatly to being fat.

Some people who are fat feel fine with their size and do not let the attitudes and prejudices of others affect them. If you are one of these folks, that's great. A healthy mental attitude goes a long way toward achieving wellness. But make sure that being fat is not causing you

health problems like diabetes, high blood pressure, or elevated cholesterol or triglyceride levels. If checkups show your health is good, then
there is no immediate cause for alarm.

As you read on in this section, please keep in mind that in no way,
shape, or form do I intend to attack folks for being fat. I simply want to
offer information that may make the critical bit of difference in consistently healthier choices. It is important to be honest about the possible
effects of obesity. Dancing around the issues for the sake of sparing
someone's feelings is dishonest and patronizing. I'd rather risk upsetting
someone with my comments than not say what needs to be said.

However, I do think it's important for you to know some things
about me as the author of this book. As my husband, relatives, and some
girlfriends have repeatedly pointed out to me, I have never been really
fat a day in my life. They know I was skinny as a child and as an adoles-
cent. I can recall being picked on and harassed for being skinny as a
child. I'm sure it's true that unless you've been fat, it's not possible for
you to know what it's like. I have learned from my patients and others in
my life that there are a host of burdens that go with being fat, such as
being frustrated and feeling like a failure when weight doesn't come off,
gaining weight despite working really hard, and hearing hurtful things
other people say to you or about you. These things can come with the
territory.

I did go through a period of time where I was overweight, and it was
due to eating too much and not exercising. My husband is a wonderful
cook, and when we first got together, I ate everything he made for me.
All of the gourmet meals at home and in restaurants really added up. I
put on 50 pounds from the time we started going out to within three
years after our wedding. It was common for us to eat a slab of steak; a
small (!) salad with rich, creamy dressing; a baked, buttery potato; and
dessert of some sort. This diet was trouble from the word go. I enjoyed
every bite I ate, and I have no regrets. Why not? At the time (mid-
1980s), I had no idea what I was doing to my health. There is no point
in beating myself up for what I did not know at the time. Now I know
better, and we have dramatically changed how we eat. We go for quality
at every meal—even when we travel.

Just after college graduation, I was injured in a car accident, and a few years of pain kept me from exercising at the level I had been used to. As a lifelong athlete (since I was 10 years old), I really missed the physical activity and probably used food as a substitute to help me feel good. The wonderful meals my husband prepared were also a way he showed me his love. Exercise always made me feel great, and at the time, my physical body couldn't handle much exercise.

Once I got the chronic pain problem resolved, I resumed my exercise habits and the pounds came off steadily and easily. I used a combination of aerobic exercise and weight training to regain and then improve on my former level of health. My focus was not weight loss; it was on feeling really good in my body and returning to my prior level of physical fitness at the same time as we learned more about nutrition and health-promoting behaviors. My husband made dramatic changes in how he cooked our meals, making them much more nutritious, higher in fiber and nutrients, lovely in appearance, and tasty.

What Do We Eat?—In many Black families, cakes, pies, cobblers, fried chicken, fried fish (really, fried anything), pork, bacon, mashed potatoes, rice, gravies, and sauces are often eaten at the same meal, giving the stomach too much work to do. Whites from the southern part of the United States share these eating habits too. But even Black families that have been in the northern parts of the United States for centuries tend to eat these heavy foods. Blacks and Whites from the southeastern United States have a greater incidence of high blood pressure and higher death rates from strokes than people in other regions of the country.[3]

Concentrated starches and concentrated proteins eaten together are more difficult to digest at the same time. Saturated fat (if it is solid at room temperature, it is a saturated fat) and simple sugars are the "foods" of the day. These same fat-rich and sugary foods are used to soothe jangled nerves, feelings of stress, or low self-esteem when unwanted emotions run high. Eating food in an attempt to get temporary relief from emotional problems is not a winning long-term strategy. This behavior hides the real problems and keeps the eater stuck in an unhealthy relationship with food and with her or his feelings.

Why Do We Overeat?—When overeating is the cause of obesity, knowledge and motivation are needed to make the necessary changes in lifestyle, food choices, and food quality to get the desired result of losing weight and keeping it off. For many people, eating is a way to meet other needs. Some people use food as a way to calm themselves, to avoid anxious or other unpleasant feelings, or to change how they feel about something right now. Food can serve as a quick fix to a longer term problem, like a Band-Aid on a hemorrhage. This approach does not deal with the core problems and prolongs the unhealthy pattern of using food as a "pick-me-up" or as a distraction. Using food as a way to fulfill other needs contributes to a sense of low self-esteem, as it is a false way to feel comfort, certainty, or pleasure.

When they feel like they're losing control in their lives, some women look to food as an element they know they can control. The thinking is that you can count on food to be there, and you can rely on having the same kind of experience time after time with food. The relationship with food is both consistent and reliable. A type of comfort can come from this relationship. Some smokers feel this way about cigarettes. I will address this attitude in chapter 9. The problem with this trap, whether food, alcohol, or cigarettes is the crutch we use, is that it reinforces isolation, low self-worth, and a sense of helplessness, as in, "It's not my fault that _____."

Whenever we believe that we have no control over how we respond to situations or events in our lives, we tell our inner self that we are powerless to change the situation. Nothing could be further from the truth. The one thing we can take charge of is what the situations and events in our lives mean to us. We are the only ones who assign this internal meaning. As soon as we admit there is a problem and change what the problem means to us, we empower our minds and spirits to come up with solutions that will work for our situations. We are capable of changing our actions as much as needed until we come up with the ideal combination for us. This is where persistence and focus really pay off.

Dieting Myths—Sometimes obesity has set in because of repeated starvation dieting that resets the body's base metabolism to a rate that is too low to burn fat. Once the base metabolic rate slows that much, it makes more fat instead of burning fat for energy. If this is the case, try as hard as a woman may, she will not lose weight, specifically fat, until she resets her base metabolism to a higher rate so that it burns fat instead of sugar. Men tend to have an easier time losing weight because they are not under the influence of estrogen, a hormone that in part tells your body to store fat instead of burn it as fuel for energy.

One of the most common confusions about obesity and weight loss is that people still think repeated starvation diets or yo-yo patterns of eating and not eating will get the results of *permanent* weight loss and fat loss. Not true. Once the body thinks it's starving, the base metabolism slows down as a protective mechanism. In fact, it slows down to a relative crawl of its former capability for survival reasons. If you were lost in the woods and had to live off of your stores of body fat, you could survive for quite a while with this slowed metabolism. Fat provides more than twice the calories and, therefore, more energy than either sugar (sugar = carbohydrate = starch) or protein does, at a ratio of 9:4:4 (read 9 calories of fat to 4 calories of protein to 4 calories of carbohydrates). Your stores of fat in your body would last you more than twice as long as either carbohydrates or proteins in this scenario.

Once the metabolism goes into fat-storage mode, it takes some work to get it back to fat-burning mode. In fat-burning mode, you can eat plenty of food; just be sure that the calories you use in activities like exercise are more than the calories you eat in your meals and snacks, and you are all set. For many women, the challenge is to find different kinds of aerobic exercise that they enjoy and then do them regularly at a level of effort that steadily burns fat. This is part of the secret to permanent weight loss. For exercise to be enjoyable, it is important that you not overdo it. Back off or stop your exercise session if you feel exhaustion, pain, or even discomfort; your body is trying to tell you something. You risk injuring yourself if you continue exercising despite these signals that something is wrong. In addition to aerobic exercise, scheduled, regular weight training really helps to burn unwanted fat. To maximize fat loss, wait one hour after exercise (aerobic or weight training) before eating food.

Fad diets, starvation plans, and the like simply do not work long term to get weight off and keep it off. Health-promoting nutrition

Causes of Obesity

- overeating
- lack of exercise
- high fat, high sugar diet
- heavy metal toxicity
- diabetes
- thyroid disorders (especially hypothyroidism)
- overacidity of bodily tissues (the body stores the toxic acids in fat tissue)
- genetics
- yo-yo dieting pattern
- repeated crash diets or starvation diets

coupled with aerobic exercise and weight training, which burn fat, are what really work, year after year after year. To date, for weight management, there are no magic pills to replace the dynamic duo of eating food that is good for you and exercising on a regular basis at a pace that burns fat instead of tearing down muscle tissue.

Use It or Lose It: Move Your Buns Around!—You don't exercise because you don't have time? Frankly, this is an excuse. As I said before, time is one of the few things we all have the same amount of; we all get 24 hours in the day, no matter what our level of education is, where we live, what we look like, or how much money we make. Time can be our friend if we use it wisely. Whenever my patients tell me they have no time to exercise or eat sensibly, I know that what they're really saying is their priorities are out of order, or they are simply overwhelmed with tasks that do not support their health. Time isn't something we find lying around out on the street like a misplaced nickel or dime. Time is a resource we all use to get the things done in our lives that we think are important. Wherever a person's priorities are, that is how they spend their time. For one week, write down how you spend your time in 10-minute increments. It is likely you will find some surprises in how you make use of your time.

Diet and exercise are discussed more extensively in chapters 4 and 5.

High Blood Pressure: The Silent Killer

In the early stages of high blood pressure, it is common for people to be unaware that their blood pressure is high; they usually say that they feel fine or they feel like they normally do. As blood pressure increases, it may go up quietly and steadily, with no apparent change in what the person experiences. This is part of why high blood pressure is often called "the silent killer"; the problem can develop and worsen without the person being aware that anything is wrong.

Then, when high blood pressure reaches dangerous levels, the person may feel sick. Frequent headaches, tiring easily, shortness of breath, skin that is clammy to the touch, sweating easily and out of proportion to the effort required by activity are common symptoms. In Blacks, another clue can be found in the whites of the eyes; they may appear bloodshot (visible burst capillaries on the white part of the eye, the "conjunctiva"). The whites of the eyes may be off color, with a slate gray or faded bluish tint.

By the time the eyes have been affected, there may have been some damage to the heart and blood vessels, and the blood pressure must come down. Otherwise, the weakest link in the system will break in response to the ever increasing blood pressure. Just as too much pressure in a water pipe can cause the pipe to burst, similar dynamics can cause rupture of blood vessels (a stroke) or damage to the heart tissue itself (a heart attack).

At least two dynamics are at play here. One is that resources, health education, and screening tests such as blood pressure checks are sometimes not as available in predominantly African American communities in the United States, and the other is that when screening tests are available, they are not fully used by the Black community. These resources are most often *not* used by members of the community due to one or more of the following reasons: lack of transportation and similar access issues, lack of awareness that these services are available, or a lingering fear that they might be harmed or experimented upon without their knowledge or consent.

I've observed that even when some African Americans have full insurance coverage, are well educated, and have high incomes, they still do not go for health checkups, physical exams, and screening tests like blood pressure checks and Pap smears. Maybe it's a sense of invincibility, a group feeling of "I'm strong, I can handle anything," that leads Black people as a group to minimize or ignore health concerns and basic health maintenance even when we have the resources to take better care of ourselves. No matter how strong we are, everyone needs help from time to time. It is OK to ask for and get help as needed. Getting help is intelligent; it does not represent a sign of weakness.

Diabetes: The Blood Sugar Connection

Diabetes significantly raises the risk of heart disease. Among Blacks, and especially Black women, having uncontrolled diabetes (either type I or type II) puts the affected person in a much higher category of risk for serious troubles if their glucose levels are not brought under control and kept there. Type II diabetes is called "adult-onset," as it typically starts later in life than Type I diabetes. Type II diabetes is much more common in the United States than type I, by approximately a 9:1 ratio. Another way to say this is that of all the people who have diabetes, 90 percent have type II (adult-onset) diabetes.

The good news is that type II diabetes is usually well controlled with appropriate nutrition, regular exercise, and stress management. If a person's glucose levels remain out of control or do not respond to proper nutritional and exercise measures, then either oral or injectable forms of insulin are typically used to get the glucose down to safe levels.

When glucose is not well regulated, it is important to use medicines such as insulin to prevent worsening of the situation and specific problems, including diabetic coma, severe hypoglycemic episodes, blindness, and other long-term complications of poorly regulated blood glucose levels.

We'll discuss diabetes in more depth in chapter 6.

Stress—Is It Worth the Price?

Stress is a silent and relentless factor in heart disease. Stress causes the heart to work harder than it needs to, without an adequate rest and recovery period. This is like burning a candle at both ends—it can't go on forever. Stress invokes the "fight or flight" response. This response can be appropriate at times, such as in a life-threatening situation that demands an instantaneous response. (For example, do you stay and fight the mugger on the street or run away as fast as you can?) However, when a person experiences stress over a period of time without a break (and the stress is upsetting), the body puts out chemicals that allow it to respond to the stress as if it were short term. Now this is an important distinction. These same chemicals, which can be life saving in a short-term life-threatening situation, are damaging if put out continuously. They give the body—especially the heart and blood vessels—a constant signal to be on alert and ready to respond to danger at a moment's notice. The body cannot relax while under the influence of these chemicals. As a result, the person has difficulty sleeping, difficulty concentrating, and a lowered sex drive. Eating patterns are disrupted, and relationships may be frazzled by the person's short temper or difficulty with concentration.

If you feel stressed most of the time in your daily life, then these chemicals are continually circulating through your body. Without physical activity, such as aerobic forms of exercise to burn off these chemicals, they continue to damage the blood vessels and cause the body (heart, organs, hormones, etc.) to work harder than necessary. This damage builds up over time, creating an environment that favors the development of high blood pressure, atherosclerosis, high cholesterol, high triglycerides, heart palpitations, dysrhythmias, arrhythmias, strokes, and heart attacks.

Each of these various aspects of heart disease is the result of a series of events that take place over a period of time. These are not problems that magically develop or happen overnight. It takes time and the right set of conditions for various aspects of heart disease to develop. Heart attacks and strokes do not just suddenly happen; the conditions that cause them build up over time.

Often the events that lead to these problems (lifestyle, stress, poor food choices, no exercise, lousy relationships) progress silently in the background, adding to the damage that is building up in the body and psyche until it finally becomes obvious in a physical crisis.

The Role of Genetics: Nature or Nurture?

When the topic of genetics and its role in health is discussed, the issues of "nurture" (the environment one grows up in) and "nature" (the genetic cards one is dealt at birth) are often part of the discussion. I think that the arguments over nature versus nurture in regards to genetic influence on human development and potential are somewhat of a moot point. Families who grow up together share the same genes *and* the same environment. They are highly likely to eat similar foods, prepare foods in similar ways, have similar exercise patterns, and learn similar emotional reaction patterns. So if heart problems run in the family, which is the bigger factor—the genes they share in common or the choices they make that impact their health? Perhaps it's more useful to focus on what you can do today to deal with any risk factors or susceptibilities (weak links in your genetic chain) by using preventive measures that address the aspects of your lifestyle that are relevant to heart health.

While genetics do play a role, clearly so does our ability to take proper care of ourselves. Both nature *and* nurture are factors in the development of heart disease. Just as we can inherit both traits we like and traits we would rather not have from our families, heart disease can be something we are susceptible to if it runs in our family. Whether or not this susceptibility, which can be thought of as the weak link in the chain, becomes full-blown disease is largely determined by our day-to-day activities—our exercise levels, nutritional habits, stress management, playtime, time for ourselves, and other lifestyle factors that affect heart health. Consider the impact of these elements in your own life. What makes sense to you?

As descendants of the peoples of sub-Saharan Africa, we are the most genetically diverse population on the planet Earth. The genetic diversity represented in the rest of humanity is less than that of this one group of people. This is interesting to note and may explain in part why there is such variation in our absorption of and response to prescription medicines and other items of the modern world. This extraordinary diversity among the ancestors of African Americans and people of modern African heritage may account for our seemingly increased sensitivity, morbidity, and mortality to many elements of industrial societies, such as toxic chemicals and nicotine.

Think of health as an investment account. We start out life with a certain amount of health assets. We either regularly invest and build the assets in our health account over time, or we neglect it and have little or no health dividends to enjoy and use later in our lives when we need them. Our health is similar to our financial situation; what we do today determines the level of health or wealth we enjoy tomorrow. We are either in the process of maintaining our health and building it ever stronger or we are in the process of destroying our health. Which health process are you using in your life right now?

Get Help

As Black women, we often take care of others. Our challenge is learning to take care of ourselves at the same time. If you're worried about a loved one's future health—who will provide care and how much care is needed—and you're attempting to find a balance between what the sick person needs and what you as a caregiver need, reach out for help. If you don't have other people to talk things over with, or if you're filled with a sense that the situation is hopeless, then the realities of the situation become magnified. Typical responses for any caregiver include stress, frustration, and a willingness to suffer in silence. These responses are understandable but not helpful.

It is critical to reach out and get help in whatever form works for you. Some folks look to their community, to their church, to friends near and far, to family members, or to hospital outpatient resources, support groups, and other outlets where information, support, and resources are available.

As Black women, we must ask for help when we need it. When serious illness, such as advanced heart disease, strikes, our outward appearance of being strong, so much admired and respected by society at large, can be a trap if we allow it to be. People may take a look at us and think we don't need help. I've had people tell me that they thought I didn't need or want help at times in my life when they knew I was dealing with some hard stuff. I was truly surprised to hear them say this. Inside I knew I wanted and needed help, and I could not imagine that I did not demonstrate or show that need outwardly. I've often heard it said that unless someone looks helpless, others are reluctant to offer help, because they assume it is not needed or welcome. It appears that help is not needed on one side and that help is not wanted on the other. In these misperceptions are missed opportunities to serve and be served.

Sometimes cutting loose and just falling apart, not having it all together, can be very healing, especially for those of us who tend to function well no matter how chaotic our lives are. Cultivating the look of helplessness can be a useful thing, if that's what it takes to get some needed and welcome help at key times in your life. Ask people around you how they determine if someone wants or needs help. Be mindful of their answers; you may find the information useful someday.

Let 'em In!

Be sure that you include your loved ones in your inner world of feelings and thoughts. Bring balance to your personal relationships; tell the people you love and trust both the good news and the troubling aspects of your life. Balance is a necessary part of healthy relationships. Do not close people out of the areas where you could use help under the pretext of not wanting to bother them. That is what true friends are for—to share with you the rich mix of life that includes the welcome and unwelcome events, experiences, and challenges.

Let people around you in, and let them know what's going on. Tell them you need and want help. If the people in your life are not used to you asking for help, you may need to spell out what you want. Allow them to help. Avoid trying to manage everything yourself and keep it all in. An "I can take it, I'm tough" attitude keeps walls around you that prevent help from getting in. Beware of telling yourself or others, "I don't want to be a bother." Bother, schmother! Get the help you need and deserve. This is no time for isolation or Superwoman patterns.

Help Comes in Many Flavors

Help comes in many forms from the simple to the complex. A listening ear (with no interruptions or unwanted advice on the part of the listener), a warm hug, a welcoming smile, meals cooked for you by someone else for a day or a weekend, a neighbor doing your laundry, or having someone else return your library books can do wonders to lighten a seemingly heavy burden. These caring gestures by other people help create the space for healing in your life. Let the love and caring flow to you, in you, and around you. Soak it up and bask in the warmth of kindness and compassion. If money is an issue, many communities have outreach programs to assist in times like these. Lots of people all over the country actively look for ways to volunteer and be of service. Most volunteers consider it a joy and privilege to help others.

Healthy and Wealthy: Make the Connection

I recently came across some information that struck me as simple and profound. For people who start out with very little, one of the key differences between people who become rich and those who remain poor is that rich people spend their time on activities that make them significant amounts of money. Poor people spend their time on things that make them little or no money. In an effort to keep their financial heads above water or simply get out of debt, poor folks mistakenly pursue working longer hours at low pay to just get the bills paid instead of pursuing activities that pay well with fewer hours of work. Herein lies the difference between working hard and working smart. Sometimes people live in areas with little or no economic opportunity. If that is the case, then treat the cause: either find ways to increase the local economic opportunities or move to another area that is thriving and can reward you with financial abundance and the time to enjoy yourself and regularly exercise.

Great relationships, another aspect of wealth and abundance, are also the result of focused love, attention, and time. There are no substitutes for this. It can't be found in a bottle or pill. Many have looked, and none have found love or happiness that way. Your heart and your spirit are nourished every time you watch the sun set, notice a pretty butterfly, hear emotionally stirring music, or gaze into the eyes of a lover. Stress, frustration, aggravation, and disappointment melt in the flow of love, whether it is sexual love, platonic friendly love, or familial love. Those stress and anger chemicals that can run the body ragged are counteracted when we are in a loving, caring, compassionate state of mind and spirit. Healing of all sorts is possible when we have emotional balance on a regular basis in our lives. Heart health, cardiovascular wellness in all its forms, thrives when our physical, spiritual, mental, and emotional selves are in harmony.

The simple pleasures of feeling a summer's breeze on your skin, savoring the beauty of a richly colored and scented flower, feeling the rippled, uneven texture of a sun-warmed brick, hearing a bird's song, or tasting the sweet, juicy goodness of a freshly picked ripe peach on a hot summer day are aspects of health and wealth available to all of us. The variety of abundance available to us in our world today is tremendous. We must all leave plenty of opportunity for this richness of life to touch our hearts, minds, and spirits. These events are a kind of nutrition for the soul.

This same connection applies to health. Those people who truly have great health in all its aspects spend time on those activities and behaviors that give them great health. They limit, or even better, eliminate activities and behaviors that do not serve them in the pursuit or maintenance of great health.

Health and wealth are two areas of life where you get what you focus on. The things you do every day, day after day, are what determine your health and wealth in the long term. Habits can help or hinder you in the pursuit of any thing you truly want.

Motivation (*desire for change*) plus knowledge (*information specific to a problem*) plus effective actions (*do what works*) equal **better health results!**

The Influence of Habits

People who are truly healthy spend their time on healthy activities like exercising, eating sensibly, enjoying sunshine and fresh air, relaxing, playing, and spending time with loved ones. People who have poor health often have habits that lead to health problems, such as a sedentary lifestyle, excessive alcohol consumption, smoking, eating poor quality foods or too much food, consuming caffeine (in soda pop, coffee, or chocolate), chronic stress in reaction to events they have no control over (poor stress management), watching lots of TV or videos, a lack of fulfilling relationships, or leaving no time for themselves.

People with poor health work as hard as anyone else, but not at the things that support and produce great health. It is as simple as that. Some of the needed changes are behavioral, and others are a matter of education and access to helpful resources.

It is hard to make changes if you don't know there is a problem and you don't know what to do about the problem once it is identified. It is my hope that this book will help identify the health problems and what to do to resolve them.

[1] American Heart Association, *1999 Heart and Stroke Statistical Update* (Dallas, Texas: American Heart Association, 1999), 13.

[2] Ibid.

[3] Ibid.

Chapter 4
Healing Foods, Harming Foods

Let your food be your medicine and your medicine be your food. Try thinking about some of your favorite African American foods this way: are they healthy, are they inherently poisonous to your heart, or does the style of preparation determine their health merits? The typical Black diet may be filled with nutritious foods, such as yams, mustard greens, and collard greens, but it's likely that the preparation of the foods harms us rather than heals us. Saturated fats, lots of sugar, oils cooked at high heats, and overall low dietary fiber contribute to heart disease, diabetes, obesity, and cancer. Cooking healthful foods in healthful ways promotes the return and maintenance of excellent health.

In this chapter, you'll find information to help you prepare and eat traditional foods in a healthful and tasty manner. One does not have to suffer to be healthy or eat boring, bland foods! I offer sample recipes and preparation instructions to stimulate your creative juices in the kitchen. You'll also find ideas on how to make various nutrition challenges, from eating out often to working irregular hours, work for you in the "Tips for Eating Healthily in the Real World" sections that appear throughout the remaining chapters. This information is intended to make healthful eating practical for most lifestyle situations. Eat to live, don't live to eat. Too many of us are digging our graves with our forks, knives, and spoons.

Culture, Food Preparation, and You

Why do we eat the way we do? What formed our collective food preferences upon our arrival in North America, and which of those preferences still influence the foods we eat today?

The peoples of West Africa that came to North America as slaves brought some of the food plants from their motherland with them. Yams, peanuts, and collard greens were part of the slaves' diet. These foods are high in nutritional value and rich in nutrients. Preparation of these foods can either maintain or destroy their nutritive values. When they're prepared in a healthful way, their natural life-giving sustenance is available to promote health. When these foods are prepared with lard, fatback, and other heavy (saturated) fats and white sugar, their natural nutritive values are greatly reduced or eliminated altogether.

The peoples of West Africa are a diverse group in many ways. They were diverse five centuries ago, and they still are today. Since most African Americans' ancestral heritage is from West Africa, the imprint of that cultural heritage shines through in the foods we prefer to eat to this day. But the details in food preparation vary from West Africa to the United States, and the food preparations by the slaves in the United States were largely determined by whatever scraps were left for the slaves to eat and whatever foods they could grow themselves where allowed and possible. Many of our cultural eating habits today come from the intersection of traditional African foods and the legacy of cooking styles from slavery times.

Food Quality

Foods typically for sale in the Black community are of poor quality. A casual comparison of the produce section and foods on the shelves of the grocery stores in many predominantly Black communities with those of affluent communities shows a big discrepancy in the overall quality of foods, especially fresh vegetables and fruits. Higher concentrations of fat, simple sugars, preservatives, artificial food colorings, and processed foods are readily available in Black and Hispanic neighborhoods.

I remember one summer day in my teens when I went to visit my boyfriend, whose family had moved to the suburbs. As my mother drove us there for a visit with him and his family, she remembered something we had forgotten for our picnic. We found a supermarket along the way to his house, so we stopped. What we saw when we went into the supermarket amazed and angered us. This chain supermarket in the suburbs, with the same name as the one in our neighborhood in Philadelphia, bore no re-semblance to the one near our home. It was well lit and clean, the produce section sparkled, and the aisles were stocked with a remarkable variety of foods. There were vegetables and fruits we'd never seen before; everything looked great, really inviting and tempting. We compared prices; things were cheaper in this suburban store, which appeared to be better staffed and more expensively decorated. As this was our first trip to the suburbs, it was a real eye-opener.

Is It Color or Is It Money?

Dollar for dollar, consumers in mostly Black neighborhoods spend more money to buy less actual nutrition. The foods these people buy do not have greater nutrition, or even the same nutrition, to offer as that rou-tinely found in affluent communities. Access to quality foods may not be so much an issue of skin color as economic class. People who live in affluent areas have greater access to fresh, healthful foods, especially fruits, vegetables, and seafood, and this means they can more easily create better nutrition right at home if they so choose. Corn dogs; giant sugary, artificially colored icy drinks; and other food items devoid of nutrition are very easy to find in lower income communities. Since Blacks are overrepresented in the lower income levels, the lack of nu-trition that is associated with low income is magnified.

Look at the advertising and marketing for food and snack items in poorer neighborhoods and areas with a higher concentration of people of color, including Blacks. Pay close attention to what is promoted and easily available. For comparison, travel to a richer neighborhood and notice what's available at the local stores and supermarkets. Observe what kinds of foods and snacks are advertised and how they are advertised.

As I observed in the suburban supermarket as a teenager, in

general, produce in higher income areas is fresh, rinsed, and attractively displayed. The store floors are clean, the aisles are well lit, and many foods are labeled and promoted as "organic," "fat-free," "low fat," "no added sugar," or "no added salt." Quality foods are easier to get in higher income neighborhoods. More effort is made inside the store to educate the customer about the elements of good nutrition. Take-home information is available on how to improve nutrition. A range of foods is available, from the very healthy to junk or nonfood.

This range of food items is lacking in poorer neighborhoods. Foods of high quality are either not available or are harder to find. Little or no effort is made in the store (through promotions, special sales, flyers, or taste demos) to educate customers about nutrition choices and their consequences—such as how high-fat and high-sugar diets increase the risks for heart disease, diabetes, or breast and colon cancers.

Unfortunately, sweet, sugary, fat-filled snacks are standard fare for many in the Black community, and they are easy to get. They require no preparation, you can just stick them in your mouth. The many quickie marts and convenience stores in less affluent areas often serve groups of people who do not have major supermarkets in their neighborhood at all. The nonfoods carried by these stores have little or no nutritional value; in fact, they rob the body of the very nutrients it needs to process the excess sugar to maintain health and prevent heart disease, diabetes, and cancer. They deplete the body of what nutrients it does have in order to process these simple sugars and poor quality fats. This easy-to-get, low-quality food directly strips the consumer of the vitamins and minerals they are already likely to be low or deficient in because the junk foods they consume don't have nutrients to give. It just doesn't work. You can't get nutrition—actual nutrients—from items sold as food that do not contain nutrients.

Eating Healthily Costs More, Right?

Many people think that eating healthily will cost them more money, take more time, and worst of all, it will taste bad too. Not true! Fresh vegetables and fruits, chosen well, can cost less than canned or frozen versions, and since the fresh ones have more nutrients, they are more filling. This means you eat less food overall. Your weight goes down while your energy goes up.

A common experience of my patients is that at first they thought the food changes I prescribed would be expensive, hard to get, and taste like cardboard. They consistently report their surprise when their food bills go down, their energy goes up, and their waistline goes in. They eat less food and feel satisfied with their meal, get full earlier, and therefore push away from the table sooner. When they add up the food bill at the end of the month, to their surprise, they discover they actually spent less on food when they made healthy choices than when they bought canned, processed, and synthetic foods.

The Killing Oils

I could write a whole book—actually several books—on the topic of cooking oils alone. Let's use this opportunity to learn how to use oils for optimal heart health. As you've read before in this book, the biggest thing you can do to benefit your own health is to be consistent. The choices you

Top 3 Reasons Why People DO NOT Eat Healthy, Quality Food

1. They think it is too hard.
2. They say it costs too much—organic produce costs more than conventionally grown produce, etc.
3. They say it takes too much time to prepare foods; it is easier to just grab some fast food and go on their way.

Top 3 Reasons Why People DO Eat Healthy, Quality Food

1. They feel great overall when they eat well.
2. They have more energy and better concentration.
3. In the big picture of life, it is cheaper than eating poorly. Consider the expense associated with illness, lost time from family, work, and enjoyable personal time.

make day to day determine your overall health more than anything else. So let's explore issues about heart health and both good and bad oils.

Reusing Cooking Oil: Recycling at Its Worst

Reusing oils for cooking represents recycling at its worst. The most extreme example of this is when oils are reused for frying. These oils become potent sources of known carcinogens—compounds that are known to cause cancer. Reused oils produce lots of "free radicals," chemicals that can damage the genetic structure of a cell, increase the generation of fatty plaques in the blood, and damage blood vessel linings (which is where these fatty plaques stick), among other harmful interactions.

I have noticed that people whose family cooking style comes from the southern United States seem most likely to have this habit of saving oils used for cooking—especially frying—and then using it to fry a new batch of food. I've seen this cooking method in both Black and White homes. This may also be a habit for folks who lived through the Great Depression in the 1930s or the domestic adjustments required during World War II in the 1940s. To this day, this generation tends to save everything—even wrapping paper and foil are saved to be reused. Of course, that's how recycling efforts were started, so that's a good thing. However, the reuse of oils that have been heated is a bad thing.

I can remember my grandmother teaching me to save the oil leftover in the frying pan and in the bottom of pot roast dishes: how to collect it and skim off crumbs and what looked like gelatin of some sort so the oil could be used again. I can still picture the pearlish color of the oil, which was solid at room temperature—a saturated fat. Now I know that this cooking habit probably contributed to my grandmother's and grandfather's heart disease and to my aunt's, uncle's, and younger cousin's cancers.

The most important thing for you to know and understand about oils is that any time you heat an oil, you destroy its nutritive value and turn it into a potent source of heart disease and cancer. Now I know some of you dear readers are wondering, "Well then, how am I supposed to cook if I can't heat up some oil when I stir-fry; cook hamburgers; fry fish, shrimp, and chicken; or leave the pot roast sitting in its own oils to soak up all that flavor? And what's wrong with doing that anyway? Food has to have flavor, and I have to keep it from sticking to the pan."

My reply: Grease is grease. It's good for your car. It's bad for your body. Your heart and blood vessels can't make good use of it. The quality of the oil is the issue.

The simplest ways to improve the health level of your meals that involve oils is to cook in ways that do not require you to add extra oil to the food as you prepare it. You can poach, broil, or bake (use a grille that lifts the food off the bottom of the pan), steam, grill, or rotisserie your foods so that any oils contained in the foods run off and are not reabsorbed by the food. If it's a stir-fry, use water to cook your food and add the sesame oil (very little, one teaspoon or less) after you turn the heat off under the food; mix it in well. This allows you to enjoy a healthier meal and still preserve good taste. You may find as you make these simple changes to your cooking techniques, any indigestion you had or sense of heaviness after a meal goes away, along with some body weight.

Cholesterol Is Not the Enemy

Did you know that all of your sex hormones are made from cholesterol? Did you know that too little cholesterol is a problem, just as too much is? Cholesterol itself is not the enemy. What your body does with cholesterol is the issue, and there is wide variability from one person to the next in the impact cholesterol has on their markers of good health.

As I've said throughout this book, balance is the key to creating good health and allowing it to blossom. The bottom line is this: Your body needs a certain amount of cholesterol so it can make needed nutrients and hormones. The right amount of cholesterol in the bloodstream is readily processed by your liver, provided that this organ it is up to the job of using the cholesterol properly. Too much cholesterol clogs up the blood, and too little leaves people vulnerable to hormonal imbalance and kidney cancer.

Butter Is Better

Butter really is better! What do I mean by that? Well, of all the saturated fats, butter is the best digested by the human gut; it contains about 5

Tips for Eating Healthily in the Real World

Everyone

Select, rinse, and slice vegetables and fruits that can be eaten as snacks and place them in containers that travel well (plastic containers or sealable plastic bags) the night before you plan to eat them. Refrigerate these food items. This should take no more than 10 minutes; if it does take more than 10 minutes, simplify what you are doing until it takes less time or delegate this task to another family member.

Another idea is to wait until the morning of the day you plan to eat this food, so the food items will be as fresh as possible. However, many people get up late and find they cannot squeeze this time out of their already hectic morning preparations. If you are one of these folks, save yourself some stress and prepare these healthful snacks the night before you will eat them. They will be waiting for you to grab before you leave your home, all ready to go.

percent milk proteins and about 95 percent fat. It also contains an ingredient called butyrate that is part of the normal nutrition for the gut lining, especially the healthy colon. The thing about butter is that it is best to use just a little; it is a saturated fat and, as such, can contribute to heart disease if too much is used. You can add it to food after it is cooked; if you do this, you'll most likely find that you use far less, as it will only be added for flavor and not to decrease the stickiness of food while it cooks.

Get Your Fiber

Foods commonly eaten by many Black women in the United States are typically salty, high in fat, fried in oils, and low in fiber, and the meats are especially fatty. Starches and sweets are eaten as quick-fix snacks instead of fresh vegetables and fruits, putting lots of sugar in the diet that just turns to fat in the body if it is not burned off right away in aerobic forms of exercise.

If you're eating a combination of fatty foods, sweets, simple starches (simple carbohydrates = sugar), and low fiber, your nutrition is high in fat, high in sugars that get turned into fat, and low in the fiber that helps regulate and limit the absorption of fats in food. This is all connected in a tight circle.

Fiber as a supplement (for example, wheat bran) is not as effective in lowering blood levels of cholesterol and triglycerides as the fiber found naturally in fresh vegetables, fruits, and whole grains. Supplemental fiber is better than no fiber at all in your diet if that's the best you can do at the time. Just get the fiber in you. This is part of why it is best to eat vegetables and fruits with the skin left on.

Fiber helps lower levels of fats in the blood and helps regulate blood levels of glucose, and it improves digestion. Fiber is particularly helpful in stimulating regular bowel movements so that the body's waste products can easily be removed. This is a great example of how a treatment for one problem can have more than one benefit.

Still Hungry?

It has been said that as Americans we are typically overfed and undernourished. I have found this to be clinically true in my work as a doctor. Eating disorders, cravings, binges, and difficulty stopping eating are all signs of the lack of true nourishment. This indicates that we eat too much food that is of poor quality and that we do not get enough nutrients from the food we eat. In an attempt to fill the nutritional void, the body craves more food, hoping to get enough nutrients from the volume of food eaten rather than from the quality of those foods.

Many Black women eat too much fast food and junk food. The nutritional value is low; the salt, fat, and sugar contents are high; and the appetite satisfaction is low. Some of us overeat in response to our body's desperate and misguided attempt to get the nutrients we need. When this happens in response to eating poor quality foods, including those high in salt, it is because we often select food sources that are incapable of meeting our need for nutrients. For people who are susceptible, salt can be a major cause for high blood pressure. African Americans, both men and women, have a much higher frequency of high blood pressure than Whites, and high salt usage is thought to be a major risk factor, along with chronic stress responses.

People are often surprised when they notice that they eat less food and feel satisfied sooner with the food they eat when they eat organic foods or food they have grown in their own gardens. These fresh foods grown in nutrient-rich soils have more nourishment to give you, and since you get what your body needs more easily, you don't need to eat lots of food to get enough nutrients. So the mechanisms that tell you it's time to stop eating (satiety) kick in earlier in the meal than you may be used to. A similar phenomena occurs after a period of extended intestinal cleansing and fasting, where people are able to notice again that their gut signals them when they are no longer hungry instead of continuing to eat until they are too full. Try this out for yourself sometime and see how it feels. You may find it easy to lose a few pounds if you stop eating as soon as you notice you are no longer hungry.

The best nutritional value and quality is typically found in organically grown foods, as they are more likely to be grown in soils that have been properly taken care of. This means that the soil is rich in minerals the plants can easily use to grow strong and healthy. These plants then can give us foods that are rich in the nutrients we need because the plant itself got the nutrients it needed to grow healthy and develop its seeds, grains, fruits, or vegetables for us to eat and enjoy. Another positive aspect of organically grown foods is that they are grown without the use of pesticides and herbicides. This greatly reduces your exposure to possibly harmful chemicals.

Although some organic produce costs more than conventionally grown produce, you usually eat less of it. It's possible that because of differences in how the produce is raised, the soils have more minerals and other nutrients to give to the plants that are grown there. Thus, bite for bite, you are getting more nutrition and therefore need to eat less than before. For some people, the decrease in total food consumption is dramatic, and often, to their surprise, food bills actually decrease because less food is eaten. Others notice that their level of health gradually improves and their doctor and health care bills go down too. The food costs they used to be accustomed to decrease as they stay well for longer periods of time. When they do get sick, they recover more quickly than was previously typical for them.

I observe over and over again that when people eat whole foods with their original nutrients and fiber intact (including fruits and vegetables with the skin on, when it is sensible to leave it on), they eat less food, are satisfied with what they eat much sooner, and have fewer or no cravings for junk food. Because they are getting the nutrients they need from their food, they do not feel the need to go on "late-night snack runs" for snacks or junk foods.

Good Food, Bad Preparation

Sometimes the foods we eat are fine, but the ways we prepare them diminish their nutrient values. Collard greens are an example of a food common to the African American diet. Collard greens are a wonderfully nutritious vegetable; they are rich in nutrients of all sorts, especially minerals and fiber. Yet these greens are frequently prepared in a way that

Tips for Eating Healthily in the Real World

Single Parents

Prepare meals for the week in batches on the weekend. Set aside either Saturday or Sunday as shopping and cooking day. Keep food shopping to less than one hour and cooking to less than two hours. Get sturdy, leak-proof containers for the foods you prepare to eliminate messes from "drippy" foods and maximize convenience. If your children are old enough, enlist their help in food preparation, including shopping, cleaning, rinsing, slicing, and dicing all food items. Work as a team as much as possible. There are at least two benefits to this approach: it eases your load, and it gives you time together working toward a common goal, namely the creation of great food to eat. These kinds of responsibilities give children a real taste of what it is like to plan, think ahead, and then act on the plan—not to mention teaching them about good nutrition in the process.

renders them unhealthy, and that's a shame. Often cooked with lard and other fatty substances, collards become a greasy affair, loaded with saturated fat, that is quite unfriendly to anyone's heart. To add insult to injury, "fatback" bacon and similar overly fatty meats are usually added to the pot to add "flavor" to the greens. These fatty items add more than flavor; they add saturated fat (the kind that causes fatty plaque to build in the blood), nitrates, nitrites (from the smoking and curing processes), and lots of salt to the greens. The saturated fat can be harmful to cardiovascular health, the nitrates and nitrites are linked to increased frequency of stomach cancer, and excess salt can raise blood pressure in those susceptible to it.

After all this, what started out as a delicious and nutritious vegetable has been transformed into a health disaster. Better preparation methods would omit the fatback all together; use turkey in its place or use seasonings and herbs to enhance the flavor. See the following recipes section for ways to prepare collards, black-eyed peas, and other cultural foods in ways that are healthy and tasty. Your taste buds don't have to suffer in order for you to eat healthy foods!

Reach for Health

Reaching for one more biscuit or one more piece of pie is not a good idea, no matter how tasty it may be. Reach instead for an apple, a carrot, a banana, a spinach salad, celery, or slices of jicama—foods that are all flavorful and good for you! You can use things like hummus—made from a chickpea (garbanzo bean)-base as a dip for your vegetables. You'll be glad you made the necessary changes as you retrain your taste buds. Your heart and blood vessels will thank you for it.

Sample recipes are provided to stimulate your creativity and taste buds when preparing meals or snacks. Food can be healthy, tasty, and easy to prepare if you know how to put it all together.

I hope these recipes provide you with some ideas on how to cook that will be very nutritious, tasty, and appealing to the eye and pocketbook at the same time. Some of the flavoring and spice substitutions are fun to explore and use in new combinations. Other substitutions are used to improve the quality of the food, such as steaming or poaching rather than frying a food in oil. Frying foods corrupts the potential nutritive value of the oil that was used for frying, depending on the type of oil, and it also adds oil to the food. All this translates to increased fat in the diet without increased nutritional elements, such as vitamins, minerals, and essential fatty acids. Fried food adds to the oxidized load of the body, and it is a potent source of free radicals that act like electromagnetic Ping-Pong balls in your body. The free radicals accelerate the aging process and also fuel degenerative disease processes by robbing you of needed electrons for repair, maintenance, and regeneration of parts of your body that need attention. Fried food is not your friend.

On the following pages, you'll find recipes for three traditional African American dishes. These recipes have been modified to greatly reduce the fat content without sacrificing flavor. Enjoy!

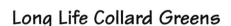

Long Life Collard Greens

This is a modified recipe for the wonderful greens that my mother and grandmother prepared for me. Time-honored traditional preparation has been modified to eliminate animal fats (particularly pork) and to enhance the flavoring with some unconventional spices. Many ingredients are the same as those used in the black-eyed pea recipes, so preparing both at once will save you time over all.

Ingredients:

3 bunches of fresh, good-looking collards (about 15 to 20 leaves)
1 medium onion, chopped
3 garlic cloves, chopped
1 jalapeño pepper, chopped (optional)

3 Tbsp. olive oil
2 bay leaves
1 tsp. crushed rosemary
1/2 tsp. ground cumin (optional)
1/2 tsp. sea salt
3 cups pure water

Preparing the collards:

1. Trim approximately one inch from the bottom of the stalks of each leaf.
2. Wash each leaf in tap water. Shake off excess water and lay flat onto a cutting board.
3. Stack four to five leaves together with stalks in alternating directions.
4. Roll the stack of leaves around their stems (should look sort of like a green cigar).
5. Hold the roll firmly and cross-cut approximately every 3/4 of an inch so that the roll falls into "rounds" of greens.
6. Cross-cut the rounds so that leaves are chopped into about one-inch rectangles.
7. Repeat until all greens are cut up. Set aside.

Step 1: Sauté Herbs

1. Heat olive oil at high heat in a large heavy pot (an eight-quart soup pot is ideal). Do not let oil smoke or burn.
2. Add bay leaves, rosemary, cumin, garlic, and jalapeño (if used). Stir and sauté.
3. After about one minute, add onions. Sauté onion slices until they are limp (about two minutes).
4. With heat still at high, add one handful of chopped greens. Stir. Wait one minute, then add another handful. Continue until a little more than half the greens are in the pot. It may get hard to stir toward the end.
5. Stir in one cup of water and all of the salt. Cover and wait three minutes. You should then be able to easily add the rest of the greens without overflowing the pot.
6. Once all of the greens are in the pot, add the remaining water and stir well.

Step 2: Finish and Simmer

Bring the pot to a boil. Cover, turn heat down, and simmer for one hour, stirring occasionally.

Makes six healthy servings. Variation: Substitute kale or mustard greens for one or two bunches of collards.

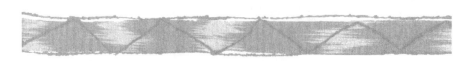

Healthy and Hearty Black-Eyed Peas

This variation on the traditional African American dish eliminates the pork, and instead incorporates just a touch of East Indian flavor. The turmeric adds flavor and color, and is an excellent anti-inflammatory for those occasional aches and pains. Many ingredients overlap those used to make the collard greens, and preparing both dishes at once will save you some time overall.

Ingredients:

3 cups dried black-eyed peas
2 quarts pure water
1 medium onion, chopped
3 garlic cloves, chopped
1 cup chopped celery (2 to 3 stalks)
1 jalapeño pepper, chopped (optional)

3 Tbsp. olive oil
2 bay leaves
2 tsp. fennel seeds
1 tsp. rosemary
2 cinnamon sticks (optional)
4 cups pure water
1 1/2 tsp. sea salt
2 tsp. ground turmeric

Night Before:

Wash the beans in tap water. Place into a large (one gallon) bowl and add two quarts of pure water. Beans will need to soak at least six hours. If you don't get to cook them before 12 hours have passed, change the water and refrigerate the soaking beans (this will prevent fermentation). In any case, cook within 48 hours.

Preparation:

1. Drain the beans. Rinse them in tap water and allow them to drain again.

Step 1: Sauté Herbs

1. Heat olive oil at high heat in a large heavy pot (a six-quart soup pot is ideal). Do not let oil smoke or burn.
2. Add bay leaves, fennel, rosemary, and garlic. Stir and sauté.

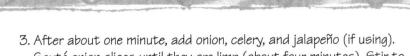

3. After about one minute, add onion, celery, and jalapeño (if using). Sauté onion slices until they are limp (about four minutes). Stir to prevent burning.
4. With heat still at high, add beans. Stir thoroughly, then quickly add all of the pure water until beans are just covered.

Step 2: Finish and Simmer
Bring the pot to a boil. Add salt, turmeric, and cinnamon sticks. Stir, cover, turn heat down, and simmer for 45 minutes (until tender), stirring occasionally.

Makes six meal-sized servings. Variation: Add one cup chopped green or red bell peppers to the sauté.

Sweet Potato (Yam) Custard
(Straight-up or for Sweet Po' Pie)

This dessert dish is always a favorite. As presented here, the nondairy mix can be used to fill prebaked pie shells, individual custard dishes, or as a simple pan full of goodness. Note that the orange-colored tuber that many folks (including me) call "sweet potatoes" are really yams and are sometimes labeled as "Jewell yams" in grocery stores. These are preferable to both "Garnet yams" and white sweet potatoes. Orange juice is a family secret, and it really adds a nice flavor to the finished dish.

Ingredients:
6 firm Jewell yams
(orange-colored "sweet
   potatoes")
4 cups pure water
2 9-inch pie shells (optional)

1 stick of butter (^{1}/2 cup)
1 cup light brown sugar

2 Tbsp. unsulphured molasses
1 tsp. vanilla flavoring
1 tsp. lemon extract (optional)
^{1}/2 cup EITHER soy milk or
   orange juice
1 ^{1}/2 tsp. ground cinnamon
^{3}/4 tsp. ground nutmeg
^{1}/4 tsp. ground cloves
3 eggs, lightly beaten

Preparation: Peel, Cut, and Cook
1. Peel the potatoes and cut in three-quarter-inch-thick rounds.
2. Place potatoes into pot (a six-quart pot is ideal) and add water to just cover.
3. Cover and simmer/steam until tender (about 20 minutes).
4. Use a colander to immediately drain (while hot).
   If you plan to use the custard to make pies, use the time while the potatoes are boiling to bake the pie shells. Most pie shells need to bake for about 20 minutes. Allow more time to mix and roll out the pastry if you decide to make pie shells from scratch.

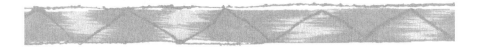

Step 1: Mash and Mix
1. Preheat oven to 375° F.
2. Place warm cooked potatoes into a large mixing bowl.
3. Add butter. Use a potato masher to mash the potatoes while mixing in the butter.
4. Add the brown sugar and molasses. Mix well using a spoon or a spatula.
5. Add the soy milk or the orange juice. Mix well. If the mixture is still hot, allow it to cool until comfortable to the touch.
6. Blend in the beaten eggs.
7. Add the spices (cinnamon, cloves, and nutmeg), vanilla, and lemon extract. Mix thoroughly.

Step 2: Fill and Bake
Transfer mix to a 9"x 13" oblong baking dish or 10 individual eight-ounce custard dishes or two prebaked pie shells. Bake at 375° F for 40 minutes. Serve warm or cool, but not hot.

Makes 10 custard servings or two nine-inch pies. Hawaiian variation: Use a six-ounce can of crushed pineapple with its juice to replace the orange juice or soy milk.

Chapter 5
Prevent Serious Heart Problems

At this point, it is important to understand some basic concepts about natural health care and naturopathic medicine before jumping into the information in this chapter on what to do to promote heart health. It's critical that you understand that the simple substitution of a natural pill for a synthetic or pharmaceutical pill isn't necessarily the goal. Lifestyle factors such as exercise and stress management determine heart health—either its presence or its absence—to a large extent. Philosophies of treatment are important in that they greatly shape and influence how decisions are made and what treatment plans are prescribed.

Currently, there is quite a bit of discussion in the health community about allopathic medicine (conventional medicine, the approach used by most medical doctors), natural medicine (naturopathic medicine, used by naturopathic physicians), and holistic/alternative complementary/integrative medicine (practiced by a wide range of practitioners, some of whom are doctors). It is important to know what the strengths and weaknesses of any particular approach are, as none of the kinds of medicine available today can do everything for everyone equally well. Chronic, degenerative disease processes tend to respond well to natural approaches, and acute, traumatic injuries tend to respond well to conventional medicine approaches. Sometimes the two models can work side by side when the doctors of different kinds of medicine can openly cooperate with each other without fear of politically motivated reprisal.

It is always wise to be an informed consumer so you can make use of the medicine best suited to your needs. If you were in a serious accident and had sustained major physical trauma, the treatments offered by conventional medicine would be appropriate and possibly lifesaving. The use of drugs and surgery are often crucial in an emergency, when a fix-it approach can mean the difference between life and death. For chronic problems and lifestyle issues, the approach of natural health care is appropriate. It offers a results-based philosophy that focuses on treating the cause(s) of the illness rather than just dealing with the symptoms.

Preventive medicine works best when it is used before serious problems set in. Once a health problem becomes serious, it takes more time and money to address, and the impact on people's lives is greater. The underlying principles of natural health care appeal to common sense. Doing the ordinary things well, day after day, on behalf of your own health can really pay off over time. Restorative medicine can be used to rebuild normal function over a period of time. You can either improve current good health or work on restoring health with the right attitude, information, and actions.

Natural health care requires your participation. It is not so much something that is done to you as it is about teaching you how to take care of yourself in ways that make sense for you as an individual. When people first get started with natural health care, they often comment on some key differences they observe from conventional medical approaches.

During an initial office visit, I often tell patients that five people can come to the clinic with the same set of symptoms, yet all five treatment plans will be different. Why is that, you ask? Although five people may have the same or different illness, it affects them each differently, as they are individuals. The details of how the illness affects them matter, as do the details of how they lead their lives. For some people, stress is a primary issue; for others, nutrition and exercise are in need of serious attention. Someone else may be reacting unfavorably to the interactions of their medications, getting all the side effects with little or no benefit from the drugs themselves. Our responses to illness are also individual and are therefore not identical. Natural health care shines in its ability to custom-fit a treatment plan to an individual patient rather than focus only on treating a disease without regard for that special combination of factors that makes each of us so distinct from one another.

In the United States, marketing and advertising emphasize quick fixes, but it is essential to recognize that serious illness usually takes time to set in; this frequently means that it will also take time for health and wellness to return. Although it may feel to an affected person like they "got sick all at once, just out of the blue," that is rarely the case. Typically, illness builds over time. As the body loses the ability to compensate, it becomes apparent to the affected person that they are ill. Recovery takes time too, as appropriate changes in lifestyle, nutrition, exercise, stress management, and relationships must be made and have a chance to take hold. Patience and discipline are key elements in the return to wellness.

Black women are seeking answers to their health questions today more than they ever have before. Most folks are looking for credible solutions and a way to think about health that is clear, personal, understandable, and doable.

Exercise

Is your key issue with exercise "finding the time to do it"? There is no such thing as "finding time"; it does not appear as discrete little lumps of stuff on the sidewalk or stuck in between sofa cushions waiting to be discovered. I know I've said this before, but time is one of the few things in life that is fair. No one gets 25 or 26 hours in their day, while someone else gets only 22 or 23 hours. We all get 24 hours. Most of us spend seven to eight hours asleep, which is one third of the day right there. A portion of the remaining two-thirds of the day is needed for personal grooming, meals, organizing tasks, and doing activities. So for exercise to be enough of a priority that you actually do it, your attitude about it is crucial. You cannot think of exercise as something you do when you find the time, because it is not going to happen regularly that way, and regular exercise is key to heart health and overall wellness.

Well, which of the reasons on page 96 resonate best with you and

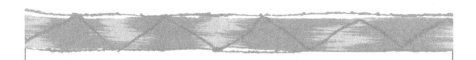

Top 3 Reasons Why People Exercise Regularly

1. They feel better overall, feel really good in their bodies, and feel better about themselves.
2. They much more easily maintain a healthy level of weight.
3. They can get more done in a day with less effort and have energy leftover for whatever else they want to do.

Top 3 Reasons Why People Exercise At All

1. It's fun.
2. They feel they are doing something to help themselves.
3. They believe in "use it or lose it" and feel they are investing in their current and future health, and/or they want to be a role model for others.

Top 3 Reasons Why People DO NOT Exercise Regularly

1. It's too hard to "find the time."
2. It hurts too much when they exercise or shortly after they stop.
3. It is not a habit, not a priority for them in their daily lives.

Top 3 Reasons Why People DO NOT Exercise At All

1. It's easier to sit still than be physically active; this is their habit.
2. They're in physical pain, are injured, or have chronic discomfort.
3. It's not part of their values and habits.

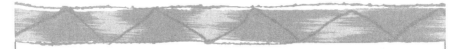

Stick-with-it Exercise Tips

Many people find it easier to make exercise a habit if they know someone else is counting on them to show up for their workout or aerobics class. Is your exercise partner flaky and letting you down? No problem. Continue to exercise on your own as you look for a new exercise buddy.

Need help on what to do, for how long, and what results you can expect? Seek out a personal trainer and get to work. Ask people whose level of physical fitness you admire to make suggestions; they may have pearls of wisdom to offer you in your quest for an optimal exercise plan.

Consider rotating different kinds of workouts or types of exercise on different days of the week or seasons of the year so you can avoid structural imbalances in your physical development or overuse and overtraining of either your muscles or joints. Overuse or overtraining can cause muscle or joint stiffness. Rotation of exercises also keeps you from getting bored, as the variety stimulates creativity in your approach to exercise.

your current habits? Keep what works for you in your current exercise habits and let go of whatever is not getting the job done.

Shift your attitude by making *you* your first priority. Then make exercise a priority for *you*. Make sure you schedule it in your daily activities so that it happens no matter what else is going on. People who think like this have no trouble making exercise a regular activity. They find it easier to get the significant things done in their lives and let go of things that are really time wasters or do not need to be done at all. If this represents new thinking for you, use it for a while and notice how much easier it is to make exercise part of your routine.

If exercise is relatively new to you, or if you are returning to exercise from a period of inactivity, start exercising gently whatever your current level of fitness. Before you begin any exercise program, check with your doctor to be sure it makes sense for you to exercise. If you are unsure of what exercise is appropriate for you, work with an expert to get an exercise program tailored to you. This personalized exercise program should allow you to reach your exercise and fitness goals in a safe and progressive manner. Keep the emphasis of the program on building upon your successes and reaching measurable, tangible goals, such as "Now I can climb two flights of stairs and still breathe easily. I am not breaking out in a cold sweat, and my heart is not pounding out of my chest."

Personal trainers, tapes, and books can be great sources of information for designing an exercise program that works for you. If you find a program that works for you right away, that's wonderful. If not, don't be discouraged. Continue to try out different types of exercise and programs until you find a few that you enjoy and can do regularly.

Keys to Exercise Success

Exercise should be aerobic, fun, and part of a regular or daily routine. Choose a form of exercise that is something you can look forward to, that you really enjoy, and will actually do. Keep your exercise simple so nothing keeps you from doing it. If exercise is complicated, you won't really do it regularly. Avoid exercise that is a "should" for you ("I should go walking"), as you'll just make excuses and not get it done, letting yourself down and destroying the positive momentum you build with regular exercise and keeping commitments to yourself.

Have fun when you exercise! No one does things routinely that they hate (unless they absolutely have to), and exercise is no different. Some people have amazingly complicated ways in which they set up their exercise routines, and this usually means that exercise is one of the things that they hardly ever get around to. Be sure that you exercise regularly and correctly. Keep it simple. If it takes you longer than 10 minutes to get ready to exercise, simplify what you are doing. That way you can get the full benefits of regular exercise without stressing yourself out through overly complicated rituals before and after exercising.

As little girls, we ran, jumped, and played with glee and zest. Imagine having an invigorating jump rope or double-Dutch jump rope session four times a week! Wouldn't that be fun? You can jump on your own or get two buddies to jump double-Dutch with you. As your stamina increases, so do the rewards of exercise. Far too many of us sit still more and more as we get older, moving about less and less until we get stiff, fat, or both. It is time to reclaim our natural enthusiasm and passion for physical activity as part of what we do each day, just like brushing our teeth or combing our hair.

As you progress in your exercise, maintain a pace during your workout that you can easily sustain. Do not work out really hard and fast, or skip the warm-up and cool-down phases of your exercise program. It is too stressful on your body, especially your heart, muscles, and joints. Exercise should never feel hard or punishing to you. If it does, you are working too hard. Feeling exhausted and breathless are signs of too much too soon. If you cannot comfortably have a conversation with someone else while exercising, decrease the intensity level of your exercise until you can. Notions of "no pain, no gain" are false. Pain is how your body tells you something is wrong. If you ignore the signals of discomfort, you risk injuring yourself, and sometimes recovery is a slow process.

A journey begins with the first step. The journey continues with the second step, then the third, and so on. All journeys have their surprises and unexpected twists and turns. To maximize the success and fulfillment you experience on your health journey, there are three key ingredients that will provide the support you need for the trip:

Celebrate wherever you have come from, as it provides the fuel and experience that lets you appreciate your choices today.

Acknowledge where you are today, as it is a place in time worth remembering and contains the seeds of change needed for positive results.

Focus on where you need to go, so you will live long and live well as you age.

Aerobic Exercise and Weight Training

What is aerobic exercise? It is exercise where your heart rate (pulse) rises and stays within a particular range—the "aerobic range"—throughout your activity. When exercising aerobically, calories burned come from fat, the most efficient source of energy our bodies have. Oxygen is used in the creation of energy while you are in the aerobic range (aerobic means "with oxygen"). The formula used to determine your aerobic range is based on a combination of your age and your heart rate: Subtract your age from the number 220 and multiply the result by 0.6 for the lower limit of your aerobic range heart rate. Subtract your age from the number 220 again, and multiply that result by 0.8 for the upper limit of your aerobic range heart rate.

(220 – your age) x 0.6 = lower limit for aerobic range heart rate (pulse)
(220 – your age) x 0.8 = upper limit for aerobic range heart rate (pulse)

The more your physical activity level and exercise program stays in the aerobic range, the more fat you burn even when you aren't working out. That's right. You can burn fat and lose weight while you sleep *if* you both regularly exercise in the aerobic range and train with weights, using either free weights or weight machines.

Always warm up properly before you begin your workout and cool down after you exercise so you feel good after your efforts. This helps prevent the symptoms of soreness, stiffness, and aches often associated with exercise. Remember, you want to be able to easily do this on a daily or alternate-day basis. To prevent risk of heart attack after strenuous exercise, keep moving around so the extra blood in your arms and legs can get back to the heart tissue itself. Do not sit down or stop abruptly after strenuous exercise, as this transition is important to allow time to balance out the distribution of blood in your body.

Why should you do both regular aerobic exercise and weight training (training and toning the muscles of the body with weight as resistance), you ask? The combination maximizes your ability to control your weight, shrink your body measurements, improve regulation of glucose (blood sugar), sleep better, improve your mood, increase blood circulation, and boost your energy level. And most people feel better when they know they are taking good care of themselves. The benefits are many.

When you do weight training regularly, you will notice that you gain strength; with regular aerobic exercise, you gain endurance and robustness. The minimum time needed to get the healthful benefits of aerobic exercise are 20-minute sessions of continuous aerobic activity; many people find it reasonable to increase the time they spend on aerobics by five minutes a week (with sessions four times a week) up to about 50 minutes. This schedule for increasing the length of time you spend on the aerobic portion of your workout allows your body to gradually adapt to the increased performance demands. The time for weight training is determined by the number of repetitions you perform for each set of strength exercises. Consult with a personal trainer for information specific to your needs and goals.

A *note about weight training:* As you put on muscle tissue or firm up the muscle tissue you already have, you may notice a period of time when your weight increases. Don't be alarmed. Muscle weighs 1.2 times as much as fat; said another way, muscle weighs 20 percent more than fat. So your weight may go up slightly while your body measurements get smaller and smaller. As your muscle tissue firms up and your body gets more toned, you will fit into smaller clothes more easily. As your levels of fitness and health increase, your concern over weight will shrink.

Many women avoid weight training due to the fear of getting big, bulky muscles. This is a common misperception. Men get big, bulky muscles because of the influence of testosterone, a hormone. Women do not normally have high enough levels of testosterone to form big, bulky muscles unless they take anabolic steroids or other drugs that can greatly increase muscle mass. So unless you are taking these potentially dangerous drugs, there is no reason to worry about getting big, bulky muscles.

Ideally, when you exercise, you'll wear a piece of equipment called a heart rate monitor, which takes your pulse while you exercise. This is a convenient way to get objective feedback on your level of exercise. It will give you valuable information about whether your exercise is in the aerobic or the anaerobic zone (defined earlier in this chapter).

If you have tried to exercise before and found it too hard to do, or felt really sore and miserable after exercising, take heart. The reason for the misery may be that you overdo it when beginning or resuming an exercise program. You may be like many people who work out in the "anaerobic" range, which is the highest heart rate (pulse) range of effort (as opposed to the aerobic, or "with oxygen" exercise where the heart rate is not as high). Prolonged activity at this level usually leaves people tired, drained, and stiff the next day. If this sounds like you, get yourself a heart rate monitor. You can tailor your training much more easily with this equipment.

Anaerobic exercise literally means you are burning energy without oxygen. To do this, your body has to burn glucose (carbohydrate) to get the quick and easy fuel required. Glucose (blood sugar) is the least efficient form of energy for the body, and it runs out the fastest. Exercise done in the anaerobic range cannot be continued for long periods of time, as the body cannot supply the needed energy for a sustained effort. A simple example of this is the difference between sprinting and long-distance running. To sprint, the runner goes at an anaerobic pace; this lets him or her go really fast for a short period of time and distance. To run a long distance, the runner goes at an aerobic pace; this means he or she runs more slowly than a sprinter but can run much for longer periods of time and distance. This is why sprinters who try to run really fast for long distances "crash" and cannot keep up that speed over a long interval.

Many of my patients are quite surprised to learn that they have been *over*working during exercise since the heart rate monitor gives them the information on their actual performance while they are doing the activity. This feedback is invaluable. It gives you a way to exercise relatively safely and enjoy the process instead of hurting yourself, having no fun, and quitting before you can get the many benefits of exercise.

No Pain, No Gain?

There is a persistent myth that exercise has to hurt to be any good. This myth is one of the reasons why so many people resist any form of exercise. No pain, no gain? Not true, not true!

Exercise done correctly and consistently is not painful, nor should it be. If you exercise and it causes you pain, seek professional help to find out what you need to do differently so you can enjoy your exercise. Sometimes all it takes are simple, specific adjustments to transform a "torture session" into a pleasurable, invigorating habit that can last you a lifetime. Be sure to stretch before and after your work out, and build in

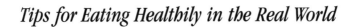

Tips for Eating Healthily in the Real World

Executives

Be sure to order simple foods or foods that have been prepared in a simple style, such as steamed vegetables, baked potatoes, or poached seafood. If the menu says the food was fried, has gravy, or has butter added, then it is not for you to eat when on the road. Why? Because you are probably sitting down most of the day, which means you will not burn off that fat; it will just float around in your blood. The lack of exercise that often accompanies business travel puts a premium on making good choices when you eat.

If you think eating something of quality will be an issue, call ahead to the restaurant and ask what foods they can prepare that will be healthful and tasty. You may be surprised at how accommodating many restaurants are in honoring these requests, as many of us choose to eat healthfully even when we go out for business reasons.

No alcohol is the best way to go with respect to your health, as alcohol is a poison. Every time you drink alcohol, some brain cells (neurons) die. Did you know that the alcohol just turns to fat unless your body can use the extra burst of sugar it produces? If you are unwilling to forgo all alcohol, limit your intake to one glass per day to minimize the physical harm done.

warm-up and cool-down phases to your training so your body can easily adjust to the demands of the activities.

Some people avoid exercise at any cost as a response to long-ago humiliations on the playground or in the school gym. Avoid letting the past keep you a prisoner, preventing you from exploring and finding exercise activities that work for you. Your present and future health depend on it. If you are surrounded by negative people, ignore them while you create the health you want for yourself.

If you want information on how to structure your workout, consider using a certified personal trainer as a resource to help you get the results you want from your exercise program. There are lots of helpful, qualified fitness experts in many communities today who are eager and ready to help you meet your fitness and health goals. Rather than reinvent the wheel, you may benefit from using outside resources. If you want help, ask for it.

Herbs and Supplements

Certain herbs and nutritional supplements have been shown to have specific beneficial effect on the heart and cardiovascular system. They support the heart and blood vessels by supplying nutrients and minerals, amino acids, and other nutritional elements that normally occur in everyday foods. The herbs and supplements suggested here often have other positive effects on the body. For the sake of clarity, the focus in this section of the book is only on what the herbs and supplements contribute to heart health and cardiovascular wellness. As you may already know, it is typical for a medicinal herb to offer multiple health benefits.

To make reading easier and help you find information more quickly, the supplements and nutritional items are grouped together according to item type. I'll talk about herbs, minerals, vitamins, and nutrients. I offer this information in the spirit of sharing knowledge, expertise, and the extensive worldwide tradition of using plants, nutrients, and minerals to better health. This information is not intended to diagnose or treat a disease. It is intended to help restore health or improve current levels of wellness. You are responsible for what you do with this information. If you are the sort of person who thinks everyone else but you is responsible for your health and misuse the following information, you are the one who misses out on the possible benefit, and you could potentially cause yourself harm. If you are the kind of person who takes your health seriously and you want to know more about how to keep health intact and take it to the next level, read on. You will probably find some distinctions that are new to you.

As I wrote this book, I had some misgivings about going into detail on topics like exercise, nutrition, herbs, minerals, and other nutrients, as there were issues about prescribing medicine for people I have never met and who were not my patients. I encourage you to investigate other sources of information that interest you. Ultimately, your health is your responsibility, and you owe it to yourself to do the right thing.

I purposely omitted an extensive section on adverse or unusual interactions between pharmaceutical drugs and botanical medicines, vitamins, minerals, and other nutrients; that topic has numerous books devoted to it. When you go to buy herbs or seek advice from your integrative health care practitioner to see if supplements might be right for you, be sure to ask questions about possible interactions with what you may already be taking. While medical doctors are knowledgeable about many things related to medicine, for most of them, their formal training and expertise on nutrition, exercise, botanical medicine, and nutritional supplements is little or none. Some pharmacists are up to date in their knowledge about these unusual or adverse interactions or have access to databases that document this information. Since new information about these interactions is becoming available daily, check with your health care provider, pharmacist, or herbalist about interactions. If you are taking any prescription medications, please check all available resources so you know if you are at risk for any adverse or unusual interactions between your pharmaceutical medicines and natural medicines.

As you read this section, you may wonder, "Where are the African herbs for heart health? Why aren't they included here?" The herbs and other nutrients I have selected for this book were chosen both for their effectiveness and their availability in this part of the world. Most of these items are likely to be found in health food stores, nutritional supplement Web sites, progressive pharmacies, and sections of stores or markets dedicated to natural supplements. I thought it would be unwise to recommend things you cannot get very easily or at all.

Note: Information in this section is provided in the format you're likely to see when you're reading labels on supplements or herbal products.

Herbs

Hawthorn (Cratageus oxycantha or Cratageus monogyna)
The medicinal properties of hawthorn are found in its berries, leaves, and blossoms. These parts contain many biologically active flavonoid

compounds that contribute to its medicinal properties and the rich red color of the berries. Flavonoids cause the deep coloration found in such fruits as cherries, grapes, blueberries, and blackberries, as well as some flowers. Hawthorn berries and flowers are rich in anthocyanidins and proanthocyanidins. Their natural chemical contents boost vitamin C levels inside cells and improve the integrity of blood vessel walls, especially the strength of the smallest blood vessels (called capillaries). Other benefits include reducing high blood pressure (through dilation of larger blood vessels such as arteries), decreasing frequency of angina attacks, keeping cholesterol from sticking to artery walls, and decreasing cholesterol levels in the blood.

For hundreds of years, hawthorn has been used as a heart tonic in Europe. Its action as a tonic herb is thought to lend support and nourishment primarily to the heart first and some benefit to the rest of the blood vessels.

Hawthorne Daily Dosage:
Standardized extract: 100–250 mg fluid extract (1:1) or $1/4$ to $1/2$ teaspoon (1–2 ml) (1 ml = 1 cc)
Dried berries or flowers: 3–5 grams or taken as a tea (1 tablespoon dried berries or flowers to 1 cup boiling water)
Tincture (1:5, alcohol base): 1–1 $1/2$ teaspoons (4–6 ml)

Gingko or Ginkgo (Ginkgo biloba)
Research has shown that this herb increases blood supply in the brain and outer areas of the body (often called peripheral circulation). One of the benefits is increased oxygen supply to tissues, especially brain and heart tissues. Gingko is known to increase the number of small blood vessels in the brain and heart, which increases the exchange of oxygen and waste products. Often promoted as an herb that can help improve memory, gingko may be helpful in situations where there is a need to increase the blood flow in the small arteries, veins, and capillaries.

Gingko grows well in a variety of climates and is a hardy tree, often planted for ornamental purposes. It is commonly known as the maidenhair tree and is the oldest living species of tree. The Chinese have used gingko for over 5,000 thousand years as a medicinal plant.

When reading labels of supplements, look for standardized amounts of 24% ginkgo *heterosides* (also called ginkgo *flavone glycosides*), 6% *terpenoids* (*ginkgolides*), and 2% *bilobalide*.

Ginkgo Daily Dosage:
Standardized extract (24% ginkgo *heterosides*, 6% *gingkolides*, 2% *bilobalide*): 40–100 mg
Concentrate (8:1, which is approximately 3.8% ginkgo *heterosides*): 400–750 mg
Dried leaves: 3–5 grams or taken as a tea (1 tablespoon dried leaves to 1 cup boiling water)
Tincture (1:5, alcohol base): 1–1 1/2 teaspoons (4–6 ml)

Garlic (Allium sativa)

This herb is used for its ability to decrease the level of fat in the blood stream. It helps to lower cholesterol and triglyceride levels. Garlic is available raw and in various processed forms. Your best choices are to eat it raw (but you'll have distinctive breath if you do!) or to take a supplement that contains garlic that was processed in some way to make it odorless. The less processing the garlic has undergone, the more effective it is likely to be in lowering cholesterol and triglycerides. The issue with breath odor after eating garlic is significant for the other people around you; if you prefer to eat it raw, consider doing it at times when you will not be around others.

Garlic also has blood-pressure-lowering properties that affect the autonomic nervous system, which is part of what responds to stress (by way of the sympathetic nervous system). If you remember the earlier discussions on stress and its effects on the body, chronic stress significantly raises the risk of high blood pressure. Under long-term stress, the level of sodium in the body rises, causing the adrenal glands to work overtime to maintain that misguided fight-or-flight response. This rise in sodium is one of the "fingerprints" of prolonged stress responses. African Americans who have high blood pressure that is sensitive to salt (sodium chloride) intake should eliminate as much stress as possible from their lives.

Read the label and look for a garlic product that contains a standardized amount of allicin, one of the active ingredients in garlic. It may also be labeled as alliin, which is what the body uses to make allicin. Look for 4,000 to 5,000 micrograms (abbreviated mcg) of allicin or 3.4% alliin (11,000 mcg) per tablet, capsule, or gelcap.

Garlic Daily Dosage:
Standardized extract: 300–400 mg (approximately equal to 4,000–5,000 mg of fresh garlic)
Fresh cloves: 3–5 whole cloves, medium sized

Horse chestnut (Aesculus hippocastanum)

This herb is used for hemorrhoids, vein diseases like phlebitis, varicose veins, and edema (swelling). It is also used as a tonic for the veins, to decrease capillary permeability and reduce a tendency to easily bruise. Escin, an active ingredient, is a potent agent against edema; the chemical comes from the seed part of the plant. Horse chestnut is also a vasoconstrictor; it narrows blood vessels and has a more pronounced effect on veins than arteries.

Caution: This herb comes from a tree that produces poisonous nuts. Do not eat horse chestnuts. They are extremely poisonous to humans! Read the herb or supplement label and look for a standardized amount of escin (sometimes spelled aescin) as 20–22% saponins. Remember: it is very important to read all supplement labels.

Horse Chestnut Daily Dosage:
Standardized extract (20–22% escin or saponins): 250–500 mg
Dried seeds: 3–5 grams or taken as a tea (1 tablespoon dried seeds to 1 cup boiling water)
Tincture (1:5, alcohol base): 1–1 1/2 teaspoons (4–6 ml)

Butcher's broom (Ruscus aculeatus)

This herb is used for hemorrhoids, varicose veins, arthritis, and as an anti-inflammatory and anti-hemorrhage agent. Butcher's broom contains two saponins whose structure resembles that of corticosteroids. Look for a standardized amount of *ruscogenins* (a member of the chemical class called *saponins*), which is one of the active ingredients in this botanical medicine.

Butcher's Broom Daily Dosage:
Standardized extract (*ruscogenins*): 400–500 mg
Dried roots and rhizome: 3–5 grams or taken as a tea (1 tablespoon dried
roots and rhizome to 1 cup boiling water)
Tincture (1:5, alcohol base): 1–1 1/2 teaspoons (4–6 ml)

Witch hazel, herbal preparation (Hamamelis virginiana)

Note: This is *not* the same thing as the liquid preparation available over
the counter at many pharmacies. That preparation is not appropriate for
consumption by mouth. Read labels carefully or ask a qualified expert if
you are not sure.

This herb is used for vein diseases like phlebitis, hemorrhoids, and
varicosities. Witch hazel is rich in tannins, which are known to shrink
hemorrhoidal tissue via their action as an astringent. Part of its
medicinal property is that it helps to tone and strengthen veins. A
vein-supporting herbal program along with a diet high in soluble fiber
and water will take away the origin of most people's hemorrhoids. These
efforts can be very helpful, as anything that promotes regular, easy
bowel movements will help to take the pressure off the veins that can
form hemorrhoids.

Caution: The tannins in witch hazel can be irritating with constant
use, so it is best to use this herb "half-time": three days on and three days
off, for example. Do not overuse this herb; more is not always better.

Herbal Witch Hazel Dosage:
Standardized extract (20–22% escin or saponins): 400–500 mg
Dried bark: 3–5 grams or taken as a tea (1 tablespoon dried bark to 1 cup
boiling water)
Tincture (1:5, alcohol base): 1–1 1/2 teaspoons (4–6 ml)

Minerals

Magnesium
Food sources of magnesium include leafy green vegetables, nuts, whole
grains, cereal made from whole grains, and seafood.[1] Magnesium directly

feeds the heart muscle, giving it one of the nutrients it uses the most. Magnesium deficiency in muscle tissue increases the risk of muscular cramping. As a single mineral, magnesium is concentrated 15 to 18 times higher in heart tissue than in the blood. Magnesium deficiency in heart tissue decreases the efficiency of heart tissue in pumping blood and increases risk of clots and blockages of heart blood vessels (heart attacks). This means the heart has to work harder to move the same amount of blood.

Just as you can't keep overrunning your budget—spending money you don't have indefinitely without consequences—the heart can't keep running well with a deficiency of nutrients, especially magnesium. Research has shown that magnesium given intravenously at the onset of a heart attack or stroke can help protect the heart from further damage and is far less expensive than the drugs typically used for the same purpose. Clinical studies have shown that people with high blood pressure are often deficient in calcium and magnesium.

Note: Excess magnesium can cause loose stools, similar to vitamin C's ability to cause loose stools when tissues have more than they need for optimal function. The reason for the loose stools? Magnesium relaxes smooth-muscle tissue, making it easier to have bowel movements.

Magnesium Daily Dosage:
400–800 mg. The forms of magnesium commonly available are magnesium aspartate, magnesium citrate, and magnesium oxide. The aspartate form appears to be better absorbed by the body.

Potassium

Common food sources of potassium include bananas, figs, dates, and apricots. If you purchase these foods in their dried form, look for unsulphured fruit. Some people are sensitive or allergic to the sulphur processing typically used when fruits are dried (it helps to preserve them for longer periods of time, thus increasing their shelf life). The same cautions apply to sulfites.

Caution: Potassium is best taken as a supplement *only* if you are taking a potassium-*wasting* diuretic (a prescription medicine given to promote excretion of excessive retained water) or other medication that enhances elimination of potassium. Too much potassium can be harmful (it can cause the heart to stop), and too little potassium can be harmful (it can cause extensive muscle cramping and interfere with normal heart function). Balance is what is needed. Unless you are taking a medication that you know is causing you to lose potassium, it is safer to use foods as your primary source for potassium so your body can absorb what it needs and excrete the extra potassium. If you perspire heavily and have muscle cramps, get some lab work done to examine your levels of magnesium, potassium, and calcium. It is possible that you may be deficient in one or more of those specific minerals.

The forms of potassium commonly available are potassium aspartate and potassium citrate.

Potassium Daily Dosage:
99 mEq (milli-equivalents) or 125 mg

Calcium
Food sources of calcium include leafy green vegetables like kale, collard greens, turnip greens, and mustard greens; seeds and seed products such as sesame seeds and tahini (sesame seed butter); and seafood such as salmon and sardines. This mineral helps to lower blood pressure. Clinical studies have shown that people with high blood pressure are often deficient in calcium and magnesium. People who have mild to moderate high blood pressure should give calcium supplementation a therapeutic trial period of three to six months or more to notice a hypertension-lowering effect. This needs to be used along with other methods to lower high blood pressure. It is not a "magic bullet" on its own, but it may be a part of what is missing in your diet. If you see no improvement in your blood pressure, consider focusing on other factors that influence your heart health.

The forms of calcium commonly available are calcium aspartate, citrate, malate, and carbonate. The aspartate and citrate forms appear to be better absorbed. The carbonate form is the least absorbed and usually the least expensive; there have been concerns over the years of possible contamination of the carbonate form with lead and other harmful substances, as calcium carbonate often comes from the shells of sea creatures such as clams and oysters.

If you are wondering where items like lead might come from, consider that a fair amount of fuel such as gasoline and diesel has been accidentally spilled into the world's oceans and that some industrial waste products are dumped into the ocean or into rivers that flow into the ocean. Much as we might like to think otherwise, it is really hard to completely escape the effects of pollution. I don't want you to be depressed by this information. I simply want you to be an informed consumer.

Calcium Daily Dosage:
300–500 mg (aspartate, citrate, malate forms); 1,000–1,200 mg (carbonate form).

Nutrients

Coenzyme Q10

Coenzyme Q_{10}, also called CoQ_{10}, is a key ingredient in the body's production of energy. Food sources include migratory fish (sardines, mackerel) and organ meats. This nutrient is used in numerous metabolic pathways, and levels of it are often low in the tissues of people with heart disease, including congestive heart failure, angina, and high blood pressure. Research has shown this nutrient to be of benefit to people with high blood pressure and other forms of heart disease. Its biochemical properties may also help prevent cancer via its antioxidative actions. Cells that are the most metabolically active are the ones that are prone to deficiency of CoQ_{10}; this includes the heart, immune system, gingiva (dental gum tissues), and the stomach lining. Coenzyme Q_{10} is found in the highest amounts in the heart, kidneys, and pancreas.

Coenzyme Q_{10} Daily Dosage:
30–100 mg

Fiber

As I mentioned earlier in the book, fiber does lots of good things for us when we consume enough in our diet to get the desired benefits. Fiber lowers cholesterol levels, regulates insulin levels in blood, and limits the damage done by too much glucose (sugar) in the blood. Fiber also promotes weight loss and improves the regularity of bowel movements if you drink enough water and other fluids throughout the day. Why does the amount of water consumed matter? The fiber absorbs the water, and this increased bulk causes the colon to expand, signaling the need to move the bowels. These kinds of basic relationships among various bodily functions really support overall health.

The most useful forms of fiber are those that naturally occur in fruits and vegetables. They are the best tolerated and most easily obtained if you are willing to eat enough vegetables and fruits every day. Focus on eating plenty of these foods—two to three servings of fruit and five to six servings of vegetables each day. Other kinds of dietary fiber that are of great benefit are the ones that have water-soluble, gel-forming fibers, such as apple pectin, ground psyllium seed husks, flaxseed, oat bran, and guar gum. Wheat bran and other cellulose fiber products are more irritating to the gut than the water-soluble, gel-forming kinds of dietary fibers.

Tip: Where sensible, eat your fruits and vegetables with the skin *on*. This is the easiest and cheapest way to get the fiber you need. Examples include apples, pears, cucumbers, potatoes, and squash—yes, eat these foods with the skin on. Don't eat citrus (orange, lemon, grapefruit, lime) skins, but the white inner part of the citrus skin/rind is good for you as it is rich in bioflavonoids such as rutin, quercetin, and isoflavones that contribute to healthy blood vessels, especially veins and capillaries.

Even though I have just said that food is the best source of fiber, I know that some of my readers are not in a place in their lives where they always eat great food (yet). So, if you must take a fiber supplement in order to get enough fiber, use this as a guideline. The most important thing overall is to get the fiber in you somehow: through foods or a supplement.

Fiber Daily Dosage:
1–2 teaspoons in 8 ounces of water, 2–3 times a day. You may add it to items like applesauce if you prefer or enjoy it more that way.

Bioflavonoids (hesperidin methylchalcone [HMC], rutin, quercetin, isoflavones, anthocyanidins, proanthocyanidins)

This group of compounds is used to improve the integrity of blood vessel walls, especially veins, and to prevent leaky blood vessel walls. It reduces capillary fragility and improves the tone of the vein walls. Some food sources include hawthorn berries, cherries, blueberries, blackberries, boysenberries, marionberries, and loganberries. These richly colored berries get their color from bioflavonoids. Quercetin is not as well absorbed when taken as a supplement as it would be if eaten in the white inner rind of a citrus fruit.

Bioflavonoids Daily Dosage:
200–600 mg

Essential Fatty Acids

The foods we eat must contain essential fatty acids, as our bodies cannot make them for us. This is an example of where the quality of foods eaten really pays off. Benefits of essential fatty acids include lower levels of cholesterol and triglycerides, prevention of inappropriate blood clotting, better recovery from pregnancy, improvement of extremely dry skin and promotion of skin moisturization from the inside, enhanced memory functions, higher energy levels, and a slowing of unexplained gradual weight gain.

Essential Fatty Acids Daily Dosage:
1–2 tablespoons or 9 gelcaps
Look for a blended oil or gelcap that contains a balanced ratio of 2:1:1 of omega-3, omega-6, and omega-9 fatty acids. These oils are usually made from a mix of oils derived from sunflower seeds, pumpkin seeds, borage flowers, flaxseeds, evening primrose, medium-chain triglycerides, sesame seeds, bran, and wheat germ. Taking large amounts of single oils such as flax oil or evening primrose oil can lead to fatty acid imbalances.

Carnitine

This nutrient is a water-soluble amino acid made from lysine (another amino acid) in the liver, brain, and kidneys. Carnitine requires cofactors such as vitamin C and iron to work properly; a deficiency of these cofactors leads to a deficiency of carnitine. It is found in most bodily tissues, with high concentrations in the heart tissue and skeletal muscle. It is required for the transport of long-chain fatty acids into the cell's main energy production powerhouses, the mitochondria.

Carnitine levels quickly decrease when the heart's supply of oxygen is lessened (as in angina and ischemia); supplementation allows the heart to make better of use of its oxygen when the oxygen supply is limited.

Added benefits include increased levels of the proportion of HDL (good cholesterol) to LDL and VLDL cholesterol and decreased levels of total cholesterol and triglycerides. Carnitine provides the most benefit concerning raising levels of HDL cholesterol in individuals who have normal total cholesterol levels but reduced levels of HDL cholesterol.

Carnitine Daily Dosage:
400–800 mg

Vitamins

Vitamin C (ascorbic acid)
This is probably one of the most famous vitamins. It is a potent antioxidant and helps maintain the structural integrity of artery walls. Vitamin C also helps prevent atherosclerosis (fatty plaque buildup in arteries). It is a necessary ingredient for normal cholesterol and fat metabolism, and it promotes normal function of platelets. Platelets can play both a positive and negative role in your blood. They allow your blood to clot in response to cuts (good) or to stick together inappropriately, forming harmful clots that could cause strokes or embolisms (bad).

Vitamin C Daily Dosage:
500–2,000 mg; since vitamin C is water soluble, you will excrete any excess your body cannot use.

Vitamin E (alpha–tocopherol)

Vitamin E is a powerful antioxidant; it helps to prevent damage to the lining of blood vessels, among many other healthy benefits, such as prevention of atherosclerosis by inhibiting the production of clots. Vitamin E also increases HDL (good) cholesterol levels.

Vitamin E Daily Dosage:
400–1,200 IU
If you are still menstruating, consider taking the lower dosage range (400–800 IU). If you are past menopause or in the midst of menopause (perimenopausal), it may be appropriate to take a higher dosage (800–1,200 IU) if you are not taking any extra estrogen medications. Vitamin E is thought to promote the formation of estrogen.

Interactions and Side Effects

There are many interactions between the chemicals that the body makes for itself and those taken in from the outside, whether those items are foods, supplements, medicines, or anything else that can be ingested. An example of a nutrient and pharmaceutical drug interaction is the effects of non-potassium-sparing diuretics on the normal potassium requirements of the body. Certain medications deplete the body of its natural potassium stores. The lost potassium must be replenished or the person may experience undesirable side effects such as heart palpitations, a worrisome symptom that may or may not mean there is a health problem. In extreme cases of deficiency, the heart can stop beating altogether. Check with the doctor that prescribed the medication and consult with your pharmacist to learn if potassium supplementation is appropriate. It always pays to ask questions.

Some antihypertensive (anti–high blood pressure) medications have impotence as a common side effect. And yes, I remember that this is a book focused on women's heart health. But impotence affects both partners in a sexual relationship, so I cover it here because this reaction can decrease the satisfaction of either or both sexual partners. There are nutrients that interact with this class of pharmaceutical drugs, and it is best to consult books devoted to this topic of drug interactions with nutrients for the latest information. Please check these references for specific information. There is not enough room in this book to go into detail here.

Lifestyle Issues

Stress Management

Stress management could be described as "letting go of stupid stuff and things that do not really matter." I often say to patients that as long as they bounce back quickly from unwelcome events in their life, it is highly likely that they will not experience severe consequences from stress. It is when you get stuck in a prolonged stress response that harm can be done to your body and spirit.

There are numerous ways to catalog personality types. One of the broadest and most common assessments of personality is to consider a person to be either type A or type B. Type A people are portrayed as more aggressive, intense, and goal oriented; type B people are portrayed as more easygoing, relaxed, and relationship oriented. Type A is known to experience more heart disease, especially high blood pressure, and type B experiences more heart health. Which type most closely describes you most of the time?

To live long and live well, you must focus on what is really important in life. Spend your precious life energy on people and activities that bring you true fulfillment. Worrying about stuff and issues that have minor consequences is simply not worth the time and energy it consumes. This useless worry, frustration, anger, and disappointment rob you of your rightful joy and enthusiasm today and tomorrow. Be vigilant about taking on other people's urgency and agendas; know what is yours to deal with and what is truly someone else's work to do.

"If you don't mind, it don't matter." How true these words are. Hanging onto old junk from your past and fears for your future simply does not serve you in living life and enjoying it fully *today*. Consider applying the five-year test to anything that you think pushes your buttons. If the impact of the issue is less than five years, let it go. You can work out the details of what needs to happen in the meantime. Whatever the hoo-ha is, it is not worth lost sleep; feeling bad; being cranky; pushing love away; increased blood pressure; a racing heart; feelings of anxiety, nervousness, or rage; or anything else that gets you all riled up with no healthy way to work it out. Deal with your problems promptly to the best of your ability, and then move on. Do not allow life circumstances to freeze your heart or cement your feet, keeping you from taking the actions that make sense on your own behalf.

Did you do something ridiculous? Clean it up. Did someone else do something ridiculous to you? Clean up your end of it and have them clean up their part of the mess. If you let this stuff linger, it can fester like an unhealed wound and turn into a really stinky, ugly mess of resentment. This festering emotional sore can transform into rot, not so much because it had to turn out that way but because it lay there neglected. The neglect allowed it to freely form associations to nearby people or recent events that were significant to you but unrelated to the upset that occurred. These people and events really had nothing to do with the upset, but it may feel otherwise.

You may begin to feel overwhelmed if you are thinking of too many things at once. It can paralyze your creativity and ability to respond in a useful manner. This signals a need to sort out all the pieces until you can once again see clearly what is in your "internal dump."

Your Internal Dump

You know what I'm talking about. It's that pile of stuff you've been letting stack up over there in the corner, slowing rotting and putrefying, stinking up everything near it. This corner of neglect is labeled "things I don't want to deal with so I think I'll just stick them over there, ignore them, and maybe they'll just go away." I don't think so. Doing the ostrich (that's right, head in the sand, fluffy butt exposed to the air for all to gaze upon) is not a helpful way to deal with people or situations you'd rather avoid.

This sort of stuff is sneaky in that it drains your energy and attention from enjoyable and rewarding activities. It can also be a source of high blood pressure that no pill can cure. Use the sequence on page 121 to deal with the stuff in your "internal dump."

Self-Esteem

Self-esteem is a valuable feeling. It helps you to keep everything in perspective and take great care of yourself. When you feel good about you, it is easy to take care of yourself and make what you need for yourself a priority. Other people want to be around you, sensing the good vibes and admiring the fact that you respect yourself. Self-esteem is a gift you can give yourself; it is a gift from the inside. Life circumstances don't have much effect on self-esteem; people with high self-esteem maintain it even when the details of their lives are less than optimal. People with low self-esteem can hang on to old bad feelings, even when their lives are going really well and there is no obvious reason for them to feel bad about themselves.

Our slave ancestors were made to feel bad by the White slave owners about everything related to being Black: the color of their skin, their hair texture, their body shape, their full lips and full hips. Remnants of that deliberate mind game reverberate today. Centuries ago, anything that was White was automatically considered to be better; that bias lives on.

When we internalize these biases and accept them as fact, they poison our spirits and sense of well-being. These harmful sayings and the feelings they represent are spiritual and mental shackles that must be thrown off in order for people with low self-esteem to reclaim their right to feel good about themselves.

If you have low self-esteem, you must also examine your part in the problem and undo any behaviors or habits that reinforce these bad feelings. Feeling good about yourself is part of the inner wealth that you keep with you wherever you go; no one can take it away from you without your permission. Don't let the knuckleheads and turkeys of life get you down; keep your good feelings about yourself for you to enjoy; share your delightful essence with the people you care about most.

In relation to self-esteem, words cannot express how pleased I am that there is much more variety in the hairstyles for Black women and Black men that are acceptable in today's culture, especially the workplace. The range of textures of our hair is dynamic, and an array of styling options has led to more creativity about our hair. We've relaxed our need to have it look only one way in order to be accepted by other

Blacks or by non-Blacks. Displaying our hair in its natural state or variations on that theme represents one aspect of self-esteem. I am not putting down anyone who processes their hair to be something else than its original texture. As long as the hairstyle choices you make reflect self-esteem—positive, head held high, and feeling good from the inside out—more power to you.

Expression of your true self in whatever ways are significant to you are part of valuing yourself at the highest levels and seeing to it that others do too. It is important to be true to yourself. Life is so much more rewarding and simpler when we go forth in honesty, integrity, and faith. Let your light shine long and bright!

Taking Care of Yourself First

No. Such a simple word, only two letters long. It can be a complete sentence. The personal power that "No" represents for women, especially Black women, is tremendous. Too many of us think we need to be everything to everybody. Despite all sorts of cultural messages and programming to the contrary, it is not true. Say "no" if a request or activity is not in your best interests. Beware of people and activities that drain you of energy and enthusiasm. What's the point of dashing in to rescue folks if it costs you your physical health and peace of mind? If your blood pressure, cholesterol, or stress levels are due in part to difficulty with saying "no," take every opportunity to exercise your right to say "no." You'll probably find it is a relief to have clear boundaries with others and to get out of the role of mother of perpetual rescue.

To get disentangled from this habitual web of rescuing others means you'll have to be firm with yourself about the importance of setting your limits. You'll need to be willing to ride out the bumps that come up in relationships, as it is likely that others who chronically see you as their personal rescuer will resent the changes. Hang in there; it's worth the work to change things around so that you get what you need. Taking care of yourself is not selfish at all. It is a wise and loving choice to make. Remember that if you ever want to really help others, you must first help yourself. It really is true.

Spring Cleaning for You

Do this process with a friend if possible. Knowing someone else is counting on you may help you avoid any tendency to procrastinate. Just like regular exercise, when we know someone is counting on us, we are more likely to get it done.

- Examine what you're holding on to in your "internal dump." Untangle whatever is in there so that each item is distinct.
- Prioritize the items you identified for completion and write them down in order of importance.
- Assign deadlines to each item by which the matter is either resolved or you permanently let it go. Closure does wonders for relaxation and stress reduction.
- Write down the deadlines; get it out of your head and onto paper. Goals are more real when they are written down and reviewed regularly.
- Post your list in at least three places where you will see it a couple of times a day: your refrigerator door, bathroom mirror, car dashboard, and computer monitor are a few ideas.
- Get busy. Go to work on these items. Methodically go through this list and get whatever needs to be done finished.
- Cross out each item as you complete it. Give yourself and your buddy acknowledgment for any progress you make.
- When you've tended to everything on the list, notice how you feel about yourself. Write down your thoughts, feelings, and experiences as you went through this process. Make special note of themes that kept popping up.
- Schedule the next time you will examine your "internal dump." This is a valuable exercise to repeat regularly until all the reasons you procrastinate have been identified and eliminated. Think of it as spring cleaning for your mind and spirit.

Until this process is either a habit or the need for it is eliminated, repeat it at least every three months for the first two years. This will encourage you to develop useful skills in dealing with things in a timely manner and in a way that is friendly to your body, mind, and spirit.

Heart Health for Black Women by Dr. Beverly Yates

Hear That Sucking Sound?

Be cautious of letting other people's urgency spill over on to you. If some-one else has failed to plan and is looking to drag you into their emergency, say "no." Don't let yourself be dragged into these kinds of rescue missions. Ever wonder why some people in your life just cannot seem to get it together? Ever notice that these very same people are usually not

Tips for Eating Healthily in the Real World

Frequent Travelers

After you check into your hotel room, visit the nearest exercise facility so you know where it is and can inspect the equipment. If time permits, make use of the exercise room right then so you can stretch and get a workout in. If you've been traveling and have been cooped up on a plane or in a car, you need an exercise break. Schedule time that day or the next day when you will do aerobic exercise for at least 30 minutes. Continue your exercise regime for the length of your visit. If you feel really tired or as if you are coming down with a cold, it is probably a better idea to rest and recover before going on with your exercise. As I have said before, balance is the key when pursuing health goals.

If the hotel doesn't have a suitable exercise area, consider going outside to exercise, if it is safe, or drive to a nearby mall and walk or run inside where there are lots of other people around. If you do not have a rental car, take a taxi or get the hotel shuttle van to take you to the nearest mall or park where it is safe to exercise; be sure to arrange for your return transportation. Many women find this a suitable strategy when traveling. It acknowledges that their personal safety is a factor, but they still get their exercise.

If you are already in decent shape, think about using the interior set of stairs at your hotel as your exercise equipment. In high-rise hotels, these sets of stairs often go 10 stories or more; what a great opportunity for continuous aerobic effort.

available to help you when you need it? Do these relationships seem un-balanced to you, or does this look normal to you?

If you are always there to come to the rescue, then there is less incentive for irresponsible people to plan ahead or be more responsible (self-sufficient). If you repeatedly step in and help in an inappropriate rescuing way, then you will be called upon again. In this dynamic, the other person involved will have missed an opportunity to learn important lessons. Pay attention to the areas of your life where the interactions leave you drained, tired, or angry. Take charge of your personal power and stop your part in the dance of frustration.

Fun and Relaxation: The Power of Play

Think of play as a way to naturally reset your stress and upset meter. Laughter, smiles, hugs, and finding the humor in things keep the heart light and carefree. Look for opportunities to have fun and blow off steam in ways that support your health. It is some of the best preventive maintenance you can do for yourself.

Quiet Time and Spiritual Renewal

Quiet time. Mmmm. Feels delicious, doesn't it?

The very words sound soothing and relaxing. If you can't remember the last time you had any quiet time, then it's been too long. In today's world, it is a must to claim quiet time and see to it that you get it. In any given day, there are numerous demands on your time and attention, both real and imaginary. If your nerves feel so jangled that even 10 minutes of quiet time seem like an eternity, carve out a minimum of 10 minutes at a time every day. Expand your quiet time gradually to a minimum of 30 minutes a day, as the human nervous system needs conscious awake time with no added stimulation. To make this clear, no added stimulation means silence—no phones ringing, pagers buzzing, cell phones beeping, or any other modern devices that can distract you from the peace you seek. An absolute "Do Not Disturb" time, just for you. If your kids keep you from getting quality quiet time, find someone to watch them or send them off on activities out of the house so you get time to yourself. If your

Games You Can Play

Card games (bid whist, pinochle, poker, war, gin rummy, and more)
Crossword puzzles
Puzzles of all sorts, whatever you enjoy
Hopscotch
Swings at the playground or in your yard
Jump rope, double-Dutch style
Word games
Board games
Hand puppets with children or adults
Trampoline—jump up and down and all around
Patty-cake (a hand-clapping game, in case you forgot)
Team sports like basketball, soccer, or volleyball
Individual sports like running, tennis, swimming, or roller-skating
   Find activities that give you joy, are fun to do, and bring a smile to your face.

children are really young or if you do not have anyone to watch them for you, consider grabbing your quiet time after you put the children to bed —if your own eyelids are still open!

If this sort of quiet time is alien to you, you may at first have difficulty in staying in the moment and notice that your mind is racing and jumping randomly about. Be patient. Just as it's a habit to do five things at the same time, it's a habit to focus on absolutely nothing for a while. One of the amazing things about this kind of habit is that it quiets the mind, soothes the spirit, and frees energy that was tied up in myriad distractions, which usually turn out to be not that important after all.

Some people use quiet time as a time of prayer; others prefer meditation, and more and more Black women are making use of both. Do whatever works for you. Meditation done regularly is very heart healthy. As the heart slows, the mind calms, and the spirit coalesces. Blood pressure is lowered during times of both prayer and meditation.

Preventing serious heart problems, as we have seen in this chapter, involves an integrated approach. By combining exercise, herbs and supplements, stress management, and caring for ourselves in body, mind, and spirit, we can minimize and perhaps even eliminate some of the causes of heart disease. The wonderful thing about this is that we're not just preventing heart problems, but we're opening ourselves in every way to a fuller, happier, healthier life. And who could not want that?

---

[1] *The Merck Manual, 17th ed.* (Rahway, New Jersey: Merck Research Laboratories/Merck & Company, 1999), 7.

Chapter 6
Diabetes and Heart Health

Uncontrolled diabetes puts Blacks, and especially Black women, at much higher risk for serious heart trouble. Glucose levels need to be brought under control and kept there.

Type I diabetes is called "childhood-onset" diabetes because it most frequently begins in childhood; it is caused by the pancreas not making and secreting enough or any insulin. If you have type I diabetes, your body does not make insulin, so you have to take insulin (by mouth or injection); type I is therefore also referred to as "insulin-dependent" diabetes.

Type II diabetes is also called "adult-onset" diabetes, as it typically starts later in life than type I diabetes. It is caused by what is called insulin resistance, where the pancreas makes and secretes insulin but the insulin is ineffective in its regulation of blood glucose levels. Type II diabetes is also referred to as "non-insulin-dependent" diabetes, although there are people with type II diabetes who take extra insulin (by mouth or injection) to help keep their glucose levels under control.

Some people have what is commonly called "brittle" diabetes. The significance of brittle diabetes is that blood levels of glucose can swing really dramatically, as if the glucose is on a roller coaster. The glucose swings are out of proportion to a person's diet, lifestyle, and exercise. People with brittle diabetes must be diligent in keeping their glucose levels under control. Strict adherence to results-oriented nutrition, stress management, and faithful exercise are key pieces of the successful treatment program, along with insulin as needed.

Type II diabetes is much more common in the United States than type I (by a ratio of approximately 9 to 1). Another way to say this is that of all the people who have diabetes, 90 to 95 percent have type II diabetes.

The good news is that type II diabetes can usually be controlled well with appropriate nutrition, regular exercise, and stress management. If a person's glucose levels remain out of control or do not respond to proper nutritional and exercise measures, then either oral or injectable forms of insulin are typically used to get the glucose down to safe levels. It is usually quite possible for someone with type II diabetes to not need insulin at all, provided that they are able to control the blood glucose levels with other measures, such as nutrition, exercise, herbs, and nutritional supplements. When glucose is not well regulated, it is important to use medicines such as insulin to prevent worsening of the situation and specific problems, such as diabetic coma.

If you are currently using insulin as part of your diabetes management plan, you should continue to do so. If you are interested in lowering the dose or weaning yourself off of insulin, *you must tell your doctor* so you can work together as a team. People with type I diabetes who make no insulin of their own, or not enough of it, need the additional insulin provided by the medicine; however, they may be able to gradually lessen the amount of insulin needed. Natural treatments can help lessen the damage done as a result of type I diabetes, but they will not eliminate the need for insulin. The current understanding is that the person with type I diabetes will need to take insulin in some form for the rest of their lives. Usually only people with type II diabetes can eventually eliminate their dependence on insulin, provided they really take care of themselves with healthy lifestyle choices, including sound nutrition, regular exercise, and good stress management habits. In some cases, type II diabetics are better served by continuing to use smaller, well-regulated amounts of insulin to keep their glucose levels tightly regulated. See the Diabetes section of Resources in the appendix if you're looking for more information on this disease.

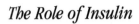

The Role of Insulin

Insulin takes glucose from your bloodstream and places it inside the cells of your body where the cells can then make energy from it or store any excess glucose as fat. Fat is the most efficient storage form of energy for our bodies. Whatever glucose you have that is not used up right away is stored as fat for future energy needs.

If you have too much insulin (either due to overmedication or eating too many simple sugars at once), then too much glucose is taken from the bloodstream at one time, leaving you tired and possibly drowsy. If you have too little insulin, then excess glucose is left in your bloodstream, where it can attach inappropriately to proteins in the blood and damage blood vessels.

Diabetes and Heart Disease

People who have diabetes are at increased risk for heart disease. Uncontrolled diabetes is the enemy of the healthy heart. Uncontrolled diabetes damages blood vessels, which decreases blood flow, nutrient delivery, and waste removal in all bodily tissues. It promotes the formation of fatty plaques in the blood that can become atherosclerosis or worsens already existing atherosclerosis. These fatty plaques can then stick to the blood vessel walls, narrowing the opening through which blood containing nutrients and waste can flow. This can lead to coronary artery disease, which means the heart will be deprived of the blood it needs for its own functioning. Diabetes also worsens other levels of fats in the blood, including cholesterol and triglycerides. In the case of cholesterol, it elevates levels of "bad" cholesterol (low-density lipoprotein and very-low-density lipoprotein, abbreviated as LDL and VLDL) and decreases levels of "good" cholesterol (high-density lipoprotein [HDL], thought to be heart friendly).

By damaging blood vessels and increasing the levels of fat circulating in the blood, what was once normal circulation gradually becomes clogged. This leads to increasing difficulty for the body to compensate for the diminished blood flow, oxygen and nutrient delivery, and metabolic waste product removal.

Normally the exchange of nutrients and wastes happens in the capillaries via the relatively slow movement of red blood cells in these tiny blood vessels. The red blood cells carry oxygen and other nutrients and exchange these nutrients in the capillaries of the body's tissues for metabolic waste products like carbon dioxide. These waste products are then carried back through the body via the veins to the lungs, where carbon dioxide is blown off; carried to the kidneys and spleen, where different kinds of filtration occur; and to the liver, where detoxification and metabolic (digestive) functions occur. These processes happen many times a minute in all the tissues of the body without our having to consciously direct the activity. Isn't it amazing what goes on in the body without our having to tell it to do so?

One of the most important things about diabetes that often is not explained very well is that the excess glucose can attach to proteins in the blood to make really large molecules (called proteoglycans) that are carried in the bloodstream. The blood vessels most affected by this are the capillaries. This process of excess glucose attaching to proteins in the blood is called "cross-linking." When a person has diabetes, if their blood sugar is not well regulated, it means that the extra glucose is in the blood for a long enough period of time that it can create these proteoglycans that can't circulate easily in the tiny capillaries. These cross-linked sugars and proteins form complexes that impair the normal flow of blood in the capillaries. The flow of nutrient-rich blood into the capillaries is compromised, and so is the flow of metabolic waste products out of the capillaries. This impedes the normal exchange of nutrients and waste products.

The tissues affected by the reduced flow of fresh blood due to the cross-linking process slowly and steadily starve for nutrients, and metabolic waste products (toxins) gradually build up until the body can no longer compensate. Once this threshold is reached, specific symptoms become apparent, and the person knows something is wrong. This cross-linking usually causes damage in the end circulation (fingers and toes, for example) of the body or where blood flow in the tissue is through microcirculation (an extensive network of tiny capillaries).

Many of the difficulties caused by diabetes are preventable or can be improved if the person with diabetes is diligent in keeping her blood sugar (glucose) under control through sensible nutrition and regular exercise. Day-to-day habits have a big impact in the severity of this illness. When brought under control with proper nutrition, exercise, and stress management, diabetes can help reinforce the need for a disciplined and regular regimen of health-supporting activities. All people, not just those with diabetes, can benefit from these measures.

Typical Symptoms of Diabetes

The areas typically affected first by diabetes are the eyes (cataracts can be a consequence), clitoris or penis, toes, feet, fingers, and hands. In the case of the eyes, there is a gradual loss of visual function that can worsen into blindness. Diabetes also causes increased susceptibility to infections, kidney disease, neuropathy (nerve damage), and retinopathy (damage to the eye's retina). Typical early symptoms of diabetes include increased thirst; frequent urination, especially at night; and unexplained fatigue. Later on, a diabetic person may experience numbness or tingling in end-circulation areas at the perimeter of the body, such as the fingers, toes, clitoris or penis, ears, and nose. Tingling or numbness is often followed by a loss of sensation. People affected this way really miss their sense of fine touch and feeling in their hands and feet, and they experience loss of sexual function (impotence) and pleasure (orgasm). Their lovers are affected by the progression of diabetic symptoms as the diabetic person's ability to perform sexually gradually recedes. These effects are not often discussed openly, yet they affect many people. If you know anyone who has had diabetes for a long time and has lost some sensitivity in their hands and feet or whose sexual satisfaction (both given and received) is waning, be considerate of the fact that this represents a loss. If it is appropriate to your relationship with the affected person and you are comfortable with the topic, or if you are the affected person, consider discussing this topic at a time when both of you can listen really well and express yourselves freely.

Giving or receiving caring attention in the form of listening can be really healing and help to break any isolation the affected people may be feeling about their sexual relationship.

Balance Your Diabetes: Nutrition, Exercise, and Herbs

Most people with diabetes respond quite well to integrated treatment approaches, such as the combination of specific nutritional plans, stress-relieving exercise programs, and supplementary herbs. Of note, some of the same advice on how to improve health and maintain wellness for a diabetic person also applies for the restoration and maintenance of heart health. Exercise, nutrition, and stress management are always your friends when it comes to health. Improvement in one area leads to benefits in other areas of your life. Pick any one area to start with, and enjoy your progress!

I have noticed that many people with diabetes do well with a diet high in fiber-rich foods, moderate amounts of protein and complex carbohydrates, and limited amounts of high-quality fat. The overlap here with heart disease is that diets high in fiber-rich foods lower levels of cholesterol, triglycerides, and LDL and VLDL cholesterol, and limited amounts of fat help lower risk of heart disease in general. This kind of nutritional plan is a good example of two-for-one treatment. Many of the problems caused or worsened by low-fiber diets are readily treated with big increases in fiber and water intake. The best benefit is obtained when the fiber comes from food instead of a supplement. If fiber out of a can is the best you can do instead of getting it from fresh vegetables and other food sources, then do what you can with what you've got. Just get the fiber in you! Always drink plenty of water and other fluids with your added fiber intake so that your bowels can move regularly. If you don't drink enough water to moisten the fiber, it will form a fibrous plug and cause constipation. Remember our ongoing theme of balance? It applies to water and fiber intake too.

There are some folks whose diabetes is resistant to management with a dietary program of high fiber, moderate complex carbohydrates and protein, and limited fat. These people usually do well on a diet of high proteins and moderate (!) fat intake, with very limited complex carbohydrates and no simple carbohydrates—less than two slices of bread or starch equivalents a day, for example. In cases like this of extreme insulin resistance, it is important to give the body plenty of fuel that burns longer, like proteins and fat, rather than carbohydrates (even complex carbohydrates) so that the insulin-glucose metabolism can be more readily managed in a tight, healthful range.

People with diabetes have to pay attention to the timing of their exercise so that they do not do it when their blood sugar is low, but regular exercise is very important for their health and well-being. Some of the benefits of exercise for the diabetic person are increased sensitivity to insulin (so he or she needs to use less insulin), milder swings in blood sugar (glucose); lowering of fats in the bloodstream, including cholesterol and triglycerides; and increased amounts of the good guy—HDL cholesterol. If the person with diabetes is obese, then exercise will also improve weight loss. Their obesity may be particularly stubborn due to their diabetes, and the insulin they have or use may be too efficient in its effect and turn most of the glucose into fat. This is especially frustrating for obese diabetics who are trying to lose weight and find their efforts do not pay off as well as they do for their nondiabetic friends.

Herbs and Diabetes

A number of herbs from around the world are helpful to diabetics. They help manage blood glucose levels, improve cellular response to insulin, or minimize long-term damage from the effects of diabetes, especially if it is poorly controlled.

Some of the most helpful herbs for diabetes are guggul (*Commiphora mukul*), bitter melon (*Momordica charantia*), bilberry (*Vaccinium myrtillus*), stevia (*Stevia rebaudiana*), fenugreek (*Trigonella foenum-graecum*), and gymnema (*Gymnema sylvestre*). Guggul and gymnema come from India, where they are used as part of the Ayurvedic herbal tradition; bitter melon originates from Africa, Asia, and South America; and bilberry is found in North America and Europe.

Gymnema (*Gymnema sylvestre*) extract, standardized to 25% gymnemic acid
Suggested Daily Dosage:
400–600 mg
Caution: Do not use if you have hypoglycemia. Glucose must be monitored if you use this herb.

Bitter melon (*Momordica charantia*) extract, standardized to 0.5% charantin
Suggested Daily Dosage:
200–400 mg

Bilberry (*Vaccinium myrtillus*) Extract, standardized to 25% anthocyanosides
Suggested Daily Dosage:
200–400 mg

Guggul (*Commiphora mukul*, also known as gum guggul) resin
Suggested Daily Dosage:
Tincture (1:3, alcohol base): 1–1 1/4 teaspoons (4–5 ml)

Stevia (*Stevia rebaudiana*) extract
Suggested Daily Dosage:
Liquid extract (water base): 5–10 drops
Tincture (1:5, alcohol base): 1–1 1/2 teaspoons (4–6 ml)

Fenugreek (*Trigonella foenum-graecum*) seeds or fiber
Suggested Daily Dosage:
Tincture (1:4, alcohol base): 1–1 1/4 teaspoons (4–5 ml)
Fiber: 2 teaspoons

Interactions and Side Effects

Be sure to ask your pharmacist, physician, nurse practitioner, physician's assistant, herbalist, or another qualified health care provider for information on any side effects to medicines that you are taking or are considering as prescription items for your use. Some drugs have special interactions with medicines for diabetes or heart disease, especially high blood pressure medications. Absolutely get information from your pharmacist on the prescription drugs you take—he or she often has access to computer databases of information on drugs, interactions, and side effects that are updated throughout the year and available to educate the public about these topics.

In today's world, many physicians are under severe time pressure, and they find it very challenging, if not impossible, to keep up with all the information on specific drugs. Everyone does the best they can, but it is tough to be an expert on all the details. Also, doctors are under time pressures to keep up in their field of expertise in terms of fulfilling requirements for continuing education and specialty certification. Make use of your pharmacist and other resources so that you know what you are taking; ask your doctor or whoever prescribed the item why it was prescribed. If any changes need to be made to your medications, discuss it with the person who prescribed the medication. Legally, he or she is the only one who can change the prescription amount or the item prescribed.

Along the same lines, it is wise to tell your doctor about other items you're taking in addition to pharmaceutical medicines, such as herbs and vitamins. If your doctor is open-minded, that's great. If not, that is unfortunate, but do not despair. It's good to tell them so they know you are pursuing other ways to improve your health. However, in general, do not expect that your medical doctor will be an expert in natural therapies, including herbs, homeopathy, and nutrition. Their conventional medical training does not go into enough depth on these kinds of treatments for them to develop sufficient expertise; often their education neglects to cover these topics at all. Medical doctors' professional scope of practice is generally drug therapy and surgery. The typical medical doctor lacks the necessary expertise to recommend or treat someone with natural therapies.

The physicians with the most robust training in natural therapies and medical sciences are naturopathic physicians. Naturopathic physicians receive extensive training in the medical sciences, such as anatomy, physiology, pathology, and laboratory diagnosis, along with academic and clinical training in nutrition, botanical medicines, homeopathy, acupuncture, exercise, prescription drugs, and outpatient surgery. Currently, approximately 15 states and U.S. territories license naturopathic medicine and naturopathic physicians. More states will join in licensing these doctors soon, since the public is voting with their feet and dollars to demand more natural approaches to their personal health care. People from all walks of life are actively seeking ways to prevent further illness and promote wellness rather than simply masking disease symptoms.

The National Nutrient Deficit

Diabetes appears in most cultures around the world and corresponds heavily with areas where the cultural nutrition is high in sugar or fat and low in fiber, vitamins, minerals, and other essential nutrients. Specifically, diabetes is most common in the parts of the world where people eat what we naturopathic physicians call the Standard American Diet, or SAD for short. This diet is bereft of adequate nutrition to promote vibrant health and wellbeing. Read labels on the foods you eat. If the food has been "enriched" or "fortified," that may mean its original nutrients were depleted to begin with and the manufacturer attempted to add them back in as part of processing the food. Commercial cereals undergo this fortification.

Check the labels of foods you commonly eat that are processed in some way; anything that you eat that did not come from a garden or a farm straight to you may have been processed or altered. It pays to know what you are consuming, as you may not be getting either the quality or quantity of nutrients you thought you were receiving when you purchased the item.

Myth: The RDA (Recommended Daily Allowance or as it is now referred to, Percent Daily Value) standards are adequate levels of specific nutrients to promote optimal health and well-being in adults.

Reality: The RDA standards are minimum levels of nutrition that supply just enough nutrients to prevent an apparent disease from too little of a nutrient or nutrients. For example, the RDA levels of vitamin C are set to prevent scurvy, not to help you avoid prolonged colds and flus or any of the other health issues vitamin C can influence in a positive way. Vitamin D levels are set to prevent rickets; vitamin B$_1$ levels are set to prevent pellagra—you get the idea. It is a common misperception that RDA standards are the optimal levels of nutrients for the population at large.

Between the depleted soils that food plants are grown in; the antibiotics, growth hormones, and estrogen that farm animals raised for human-consumption are fed; and RDA levels that represent minimal levels of nutrition, a person with diabetes would do well to take supplements that round out whatever they may be missing from their nutritional sources. While I am not a big fan of popping pills all day (be they natural, synthetic, or pharmaceutical), I also recognize that we live in a world where we cannot take it for granted that we will get enough nutrients in our diet if we ignore our intake levels. Read books that address these issues and seek the help of qualified heath professionals in deciding what makes sense for your supplementation needs. There are labs that can tell you and your health care provider objectively what nutrients you are deficient in, what nutrients you may not digest or metabolize and absorb well, if your bodily usage and storage are adequate, or even if you have an excess of a particular nutrient or nutrients. Some nutrients are best measured in the blood, urine, saliva, or stool, depending on where they are the most stable or where the markers of their metabolism are most accurate. It is a good idea to get some objective measurement of your nutrient status.

Remember the Unholy Trio?

Out-of-control diabetes is part of the "unholy trio" discussed in chapter 3. The other elements of this unholy trio are high blood pressure and obesity. These three factors combined really put Black women over the edge for risk of heart disease, especially severe forms of heart disease. Since the overwhelming majority of diabetes is type II (adult-onset or insulin-resistant) and not type I (insulin-dependent), this means that much of the possible harm can be prevented.

Taming this unholy trio is possible, as all three elements—uncontrolled diabetes, high blood pressure, and obesity—can be managed or improved with the use of elements in the toolbox of natural health care, such as nutrition, exercise, and stress management. These everyday choices put the power to promote better health in the hands of the person who would most benefit from it—the person who wants to make the needed changes and does what is necessary to get the results they seek. That person is you!

Chapter 7
The Price of Silence

What price silence? Keeping the truth about how we really feel to ourselves may be a trait left over from the legacy of slavery, a time when there was little opportunity for open expressions of feelings, let alone possible symptoms. The slaves received very little or no medical care, so even if they did say they thought something was wrong, it was not likely to be heard and acted upon by anyone who could offer help.

Use of centuries-old African healing and medical traditions continued as the slaves tried to make the best of a bad situation. Members of the slave communities who had skills in the healing arts were sought when the need arose. The harshness of the slaves' lives and the fact that they were frequently sold and forced to move around meant that there were real obstacles to passing on all of the healing knowledge and traditions these people brought with them to North America.

Communication about our health is key. If we're not talking about our health issues, the next generation has little or no idea of what may await them with respect to their health. If this is the case, neither prevention of illness nor the consequences of disease can be successfully addressed. The health care you're seeking is made less effective if your health care provider is unaware of your risk factors, simply because family members did not talk openly about their health and in enough detail to be useful. Sometimes folks withhold information, especially what they may perceive as negative or unpleasant information, because they think that this knowledge will somehow be a bother to the person hearing it. It is often said in the Black community that older folks keep a lot to themselves, and the family health history is one of those areas that typically does not get passed down for younger folks to know. One of the many things I appreciate about my mother is that she has always made the effort to tell me about her health and whatever she remembered about my grandparents' health. Her intention is that I know about possible family susceptibilities so I can focus on prevention around specific issues.

African American people historically have had inadequate health care and limited access to health care. As I wrote this book, numerous health care professionals asked why Black women and men do not participate more actively in health screenings, free blood pressure checks, and other community outreach efforts. My response, as I noted in chapter 3, was that several issues are at work. Some of the lack of participation is due to mistrust of White health care professionals in general; some of it is due to health not being a top priority; some of it is due to not knowing these services are available and that regular checkups are important; and finally, a portion of this is due to inability to travel to health care facilities. If the person does not have a car or someone who can drive for them, cab fare can be prohibitively expensive. (These factors are discussed in more depth in chapters 2 and 3.)

Whatever the reasons may be, the only people we hurt are ourselves when we do not take full advantage of health-related services available in our communities or workplaces. Problems like high blood pressure can be simple to keep under control or eliminate completely when caught early on and promptly treated. If neglected, these kinds of health problems can become more severe over time. They can keep us from the life activities we thought we'd enjoy forever and place more work on the shoulders of those who must take care of us when we can no longer do things for ourselves.

Knowledge is power. Keep your loved ones out of the dark by shining the light of information concerning your health on them. Take the time to catalog and record your family's health history as best you can. Interview older members of the family. Learn what they remember about family health and illness. If they do not know particular disease names, then take a good guess at them by listing any complaints the person had or things about their appearance that might be clues, such as a hump back, an amputation, shortness of breath, and lots of veins on the surface of their legs. These clues provide helpful information on the health status of family members who, for whatever reasons, may not be able to tell you directly about their health. My father is in the middle of a project to collect data from family members about when their diabetes started. His intention is to share the information with the following generations so they will know what to watch for and the importance of getting help early. Perhaps there's someone in your family who'd be interested in taking on a project like this to better inform family members and encourage open communication.

Because we African Americans tend to not talk about our health in much detail, even with loved ones, family members and friends often have no idea that someone they know and love is ill or that the person they care about is experiencing odd sensations and outright symptoms of disease. The seriousness of the illness seems to not be much of a factor, as folks can be just as reluctant to say they are having a bad bout of hay fever as they are to tell others that they have cancer. Some folks prefer the certainty of silence over taking a chance on how other people in their lives will respond to the news.

Children and grandchildren often have no clue about the health of their parents and grandparents. They may notice decreases in activity levels, fewer interests, or reduced mobility and wonder if everything is all right. When the elder is asked, a typical response is something like "I'm OK, I just feel a bit under the weather," regardless of how good or bad she or he really feels. It is normal that different people express themselves in different ways. The problem comes when key information is omitted. This omission shuts out potential sources of help, including appropriate treatment and tender loving care.

This silence reinforces a needless sense of mystery concerning medicine and health care. The younger members of the family are often not clear on what illnesses others in their family had, and so they don't know what they are at risk for themselves. This is sad and unnecessary.

Tips for Eating Healthily in the Real World

If You Eat out Often

Many foods prepared in restaurants and fast food chains are high in salt, fat, and sugar. That has a lot to do with why our jaded taste buds often enjoy eating out so much. Avoid salty items on the menu, such as anything you know has to be salted as a key part of its preparation; smoked or cured meats are a great example of this. Do not eat foods high in fat, such as fried anything; fettuccine Alfredo; white sauces; creams; gravies; white chocolate (it's all fat!); buttery, sugary items; and meats baked in their own juices, which means melted fat from the meat. Meat prepared this way also reabsorbs some of the fat. Shift your choices toward salads with simple dressings, steamed or broiled vegetables, potatoes with the skin on, brown rice (more fiber than white rice), or wild rice (even higher fiber content), and fish and meat that are poached, grilled, or broiled.

There is so much more information available today on health in bookstores, libraries, the Internet, magazines, television, and other media outlets. Suffering in silence or ignorance just doesn't make sense. We need to talk to each other honestly about how we feel, what we experience, and the impact it has in our lives.

I know of a situation where a Black woman had cancer and insisted that no one outside of her immediate family be told. The week before she died, lifelong friends were finally told the news. They were shocked, afraid they would lose her quickly, and angry that they were not told sooner as they wanted to help, if possible. I recognize that it is up to each person to handle their private information as they best see fit. However, I advocate a balance between privacy and sharing important information with loved ones. If you decide not to share the news about your illness with others, understand that you may be increasing the emotional and psychological isolation that you experience. This kind of isolation is not healing.

I know of a different situation where an entire generation of 13 siblings has diabetes mellitus; one had type I (childhood-onset) diabetes, and the rest had or have type II diabetes. It is remarkable that all of the siblings of such a large family have diabetes in one form or another. The family response to this situation is heartening, given the context of folks not opening up and sharing what is really going on with their health. Like my father in our family, one of the elder brothers is gathering information on the impact of the illness and the treatments being used so it can be shared with the younger members of the family. Prevention is the key here, and it could make a big difference in the quantity and quality of life these people enjoy.

Adoptees and Health Records

Adoptees face a special situation concerning their health heritage. In some states, it is illegal or practically impossible for them to acquire the health records of their birth parents because of confidentiality laws concerning the right of birth parents to remain anonymous. Some states are more progressive concerning this issue than others.

Having had a number of adoptees as patients and having run right smack into this issue with them, I can say how frustrating it is to not be able to be more specific concerning their risks for any particular illness. This situation forces a focus on the "nurture" or lifestyle and environmental aspects of health because information on the "nature" or genetic aspect is unavailable. It is my hope that someday soon all adoptees will be able to get information on their parents' medical history, while the birth parents' identity remains confidential. When this happens, vital medical and genetic history will be shared even as privacy is preserved.

When trying to be of service to a patient and make an accurate health assessment, a doctor or any other kind of health provider needs to know what someone is at risk for. The absence of this information really lessens the accuracy of the health risk assessment. For adoptees, this means they lose out through no fault of their own. While life is not always fair, it is best to remove unneeded bias and confusion where possible. In the case of adoptees and access to family medical histories, this is an obvious opportunity for clarity and truth.

The Hidden Costs of Heart Disease

There are the obvious costs—financial and other—of illness of any sort, including heart diseases of various kinds. Little discussed, and unfortunately frequently experienced, are the hidden costs of heart disease. The quality of life for people with moderate to severe heart disease goes steadily downhill, including an ever dwindling list of activities they can safely and comfortably participate in.

The impact for the person's family and friends is just as significant, especially if they are also caregivers for the affected person. The losses can be widespread: loss of fun times, inability to participate in activities that involve physical exertion, dulling or loss of mental abilities, loss of connection with loved ones. For example, strokes can alter people's abili-

---

Tips for Eating Healthily in the Real World

Shift Work or Irregular Work Hours

If you are hungry at the end of your shift and plan to eat a large meal shortly before going to bed, don't do it. Eating right before going to sleep puts a strain on your digestion and your heart. This isn't good. If bedtime is less than three hours away, skip the large meal. Make a different choice. If you feel you cannot go to sleep without eating something, make yourself a fruit smoothie. Use a blender to combine a banana with pineapple juice or soy milk, as well as some strawberries or blueberries, or combine apple juice and a banana. If that's not your cup of tea, so to speak, have some freshly made vegetable juice (parsley, celery, carrots, cucumber, and ginger root) instead. It will satisfy your hunger and it is quickly digested, avoiding an episode of heartburn while you are trying to get some much-needed rest. The smoothie and the fresh juice are rich in nutrients and quite tasty too. An added bonus is that they take less than five minutes to prepare—a real benefit when you are tired at the end of your work day. You can add powdered spirulina or fiber for additional health benefits.

ties to express themselves as well as affect their personality, their mobility, and their judgment. If a person does not fully recover from a stroke, family members and friends miss the person they knew before the stroke occurred.

Folks just plain feel bad when they have high blood pressure or the complications of heart disease. They are not as active as they want to be and usually miss their former level of social activity and physical ability. Not feeling well interferes with relationships, a personal sense of well-being, job performance, and family obligations. Other people in their life miss the activities and other aspects of living that were shared when the person was relatively well. The result is a loss for everyone involved.

With knowledge of prevention, all of this loss can be avoided. Some people do not value prevention, thinking of it as something for someone else to do or benefit from. We have so much information today about health that our choices are clear. It is up to you to take the needed steps for prevention to work in your life. Choosing to ignore preventive measures is foolish. You need to understand, too, that if you make a conscious choice to avoid prevention despite now knowing what preventive steps to take in your life, you'll achieve the same results as ignorance. These choices are all yours to make.

If you choose to make wise decisions about your health and take prevention seriously, congratulations! Your efforts will reward you throughout your lifetime. If you ignore preventive measures and disaster strikes, you need to take ownership of what has happened. You can only change the things in your life that you take responsibility and accountability for. Share what you have learned with others who are willing to listen and learn from your mistakes. You may help someone else you know avoid a health catastrophe.

Chapter 8
Is Estrogen Replacement Therapy Protective?

Hormones: They are in the news on an almost daily basis. The public is bombarded with reports about the effect of too many hormones in things like beef and chicken. At the same time, much information is presented concerning a relative lack of hormones, especially for women after menopause. Wading through the multitude of conflicting opinions to find something meaningful can be nearly impossible. Besides, how do we know whether the slough of information about women and hormones applies equally to all women, not just White women—the group of women most frequently studied in the United States?

When considering hormone use for any reason, such as to replenish an actual deficiency or to quench an excess of a particular hormone, balance is the key. This point cannot be overemphasized.

Hormones are powerful substances in our bodies. They're biochemical marvels, really, because a tiny amount can have a big effect. The use of such powerful chemicals for any reason must be carefully weighed against all risk factors before making a decision about their use.

First Heart Attacks Kill Women More Often than Men

Recent research has shown that women are more likely than men to die from their first heart attack.[1] This is puzzling to many of my patients, and frankly, it's puzzling to some doctors. Many people do not have it in their minds that women after menopause have the same *risk* for heart disease as men, even though the *incidence* does not quite catch up to that in men. What's more, recent research has also shown that first-time heart attacks are also more deadly in younger women, who have not reached menopause, than in younger men. Americans often don't associate heart disease with women, and because of this, women who have it may not recognize the symptoms for what they are and get help accordingly. Some people in the medical community still believe that men get heart disease and women don't get it as much or as severely, which is false. Some studies showed that doctors did not perform the more aggressive or invasive procedures, treatments, and tests on their female patients as often as they did for their male patients.

Now that we know about our increased risk for heart disease after menopause, women can and should ask better questions concerning their heart health. Recognizing you have a problem and getting prompt treatment are keys to keeping heart disease from being deadly.

In the coming years, further areas of enlightenment in medicine will unfold. The pendulum will swing back—something that was once thought to be true will be discovered as false, and new thinking will occur on that topic. This is a normal and welcome process in the world of science, where old knowledge, ignorance, and misunderstanding are replaced by the latest thinking.

Menopause, Estrogen, and Heart Health

Menopause is a natural and normal phase in a woman's life cycle. It is not a disease. Menopause is technically defined as the time of the last menstrual cycle. Perimenopause refers to the time around actual menopause when a woman's cycle may begin to change, becoming more or less frequent before it stops altogether. Her pattern of bleeding may increase or decrease, and her sense of herself may shift as her reproductive capacity comes to an end. Many heterosexual women experience relief about not having to worry about contraception anymore. They find they have a stronger sense of self after menopause coupled with greater clarity about who they are as people and what they want from life.

Menopause is a time when expectations become self-fulfilling. Women who expect a fairly smooth experience usually have one, and those who think it will be hard are more likely to experience significant difficulties. Numerous studies of various cultures around the world show that when the women expect menopause to be straightforward, it usually is, and when they believe that menopause means the female body is falling apart, they much more often have major problems.

The current efforts to transform menopause into a disease entity are driven by the desire to sell stuff to women by making them think that menopause is a problem. Many women go through menopause without any major complaints. Some even have such a smooth experience that the only clue they have to signal them that they're experiencing menopause is that their menstrual cycle has stopped—no hot flashes, no drenching sweats, no wild mood swings, no insomnia, no other troublesome complaints occasionally associated with menopause. At this time, it appears that among the world's women, White women are the most likely to have problems with the transition of life that menopause represents.

Menopause is a normal part of a woman's life cycle—it is a universal experience for women around the world, provided they live long enough to reach it. Menopause is experienced regardless of a woman's race, economic status, education level, or belief system.

Part of the reality of menopause is that there is a significant decrease in both the estrogen and progesterone produced by the body. This is a normal event; the higher amounts of estrogen and progesterone are required by the body for reproduction. Since it is normal for levels of these hormones to decrease after menopause, is it wise to add them back via drugs, in the form of hormone replacement therapy, regardless of whether they are natural or synthetic?

There are risks associated with excess estrogen over a woman's lifetime, namely increased risk of cancer of the breast, ovaries, and uterus (actually the uterine lining, the endometrium). Progesterone should usually be prescribed along with estrogen if a woman still has her uterus or ovaries. When estrogen is prescribed alone, it is referred to as "unopposed estrogen," because it is typical for larger amounts of estrogen to appear in a woman's body at the same time as significant amounts of progesterone as part of her natural hormonal cycle before menopause. It may be OK to give estrogen alone if a woman has had a total hysterectomy, since the risk of ovarian or uterine cancer is gone (although the risk for breast cancer remains). Given these risks, the most important question women and their health care practitioners need to answer is: Is there a big enough benefit to heart health from replacing estrogen in order to justify these risks? Does it make sense to give a woman estrogen after menopause to protect her against heart disease? Weigh the trade-off of presumed heart protection from taking estrogen against the already established increased risk of cancers of the breast, uterus, and ovaries due to prolonged excess estrogen exposure.

Does Estrogen Decrease the Risk for Heart Disease?

The newest findings about a woman's increased risk for heart disease after menopause led to the hypothesis that perhaps the difference in heart disease rates between men and women was due to the influence of estrogen in women's physiology. Since estrogen is a vasodilator of coronary arteries, it can widen the arteries that feed blood to the heart tissue. Women have significant amounts of estrogen in their bodies, while men have very little.

Some health care practitioners have wondered, why not consider progesterone, testosterone, pregnenolone, androstenedione, DHEA, or any other hormones as possible sources of protection from heart disease? Why just look at estrogen? These are good questions. When thinking about hormones, it is useful to keep in mind my ongoing theme of balance and consider whether the issues of excess, deficiency, or normal amounts are relevant to this issue.

For example, progesterone, in some forms, can counteract the heart-friendly benefit that estrogen offers some women. Progesterone's effect when taken alone or in combination with estrogen needs more research done over a longer time before we can really be sure of its effect on heart health. When taken as a medicine, progesterone is available in different forms; micronized progesterone (this means it is crushed and suspended in tiny pieces so it is more easily absorbed) seems to counteract the positive effect estrogen can have on the heart the least. Progestins (a different form of progesterone) interfere with the heart-healthy benefit of estrogen to varying degrees.

If you are at risk for or have coronary artery disease, estrogen therapy can be beneficial in reducing the risk of a first-time heart attack or repeated episodes. Given that it is normal and natural for estrogen to greatly decrease in a woman's body after menopause, the only way to get the estrogen after menopause is through some kind of supplementation, whether it is pharmaceutical, plant based, from your own fat stores, or some other yet to be discovered source. It is possible that taking estrogen to help protect the heart helps to hide other factors that increase women's risk for heart disease after menopause. The best possible strategy is to eat really well, exercise regularly, keep stress at low levels, and harvest the bounty of fulfilling relationships in your life. If these factors that affect heart health are covered, it doesn't seem to make sense to give a woman extra estrogen unless she is at high risk for osteoporosis and is not at high risk for cancers of the uterus, breast, and ovaries.

As part of the larger perspective, it is important to remember that sooner or later every one dies of heart failure, loosely defined. Once the heart stops beating, you die. So the latest hubbub about women, estrogen, and heart disease needs to be considered in the larger context of what is really affecting the heart disease statistics, especially for African American women. It could be more fruitful to focus on regular exercise, sound nutrition, stress reduction, and fulfilling relationships than to em-phasize estrogen as a stand-alone treatment and preventive agent for heart disease, especially coronary artery disease.

Does Estrogen Replacement Therapy Make Sense for the Typical Black Woman?

In specific cases, yes. The greatest protection from estrogen replacement therapy (ERT) goes to women who have high risk for, or who currently have, heart disease. Estrogen can dilate narrowed coronary arteries, the arteries that carry blood to the heart itself. For most women, including Black women, if there is no risk for coronary artery disease or existing coronary artery disease, then ERT does not make sense. It is far better to make wise choices about nutrition, exercise, and stress management than to indefinitely pop a pill that can increase your risk of estrogen-sensitive cancers. Now let me share with you the reasons why I say this.

There is no such thing as one-size-fits-all health advice. With that in mind, I want to explore some of the issues likely to be sources of either confusion or concern for Black women around the topic of ERT. It is important to clarify these points because today, much of the discussion for women concerning estrogen centers on either avoiding osteoporosis or preventing serious heart disease after menopause. The physiologic transition brought on by menopause changes the body's amount of estrogen and progesterone, the predominant hormones that affect women's lives from puberty to menopause. These significant hormones play an important role in reproductive health, childbearing, and an overall sense of well-being.

Some women feel that after menopause, it doesn't make any sense to replace what nature purposely had drop off; they oppose estrogen or other hormone replacement therapy because they think it interferes with the natural rhythm of life. After a woman stops having her menstrual period, her body produces relatively little estrogen. For many women, this means that her breasts are no longer sore or tender, but her vaginal tissue may be drier and wrinkles on her skin may become more pronounced.

To explore whether ERT makes sense, all the factors that go into the overall decision must be understood. In these next sections, I focus on the factors that are more likely to affect you.

Black Women, Obesity, and Estrogen

We've already established that Black women are overrepresented among overweight Americans. In fact, we as a group are the most overweight and the most obese. While there's no need to flip to the other side and become anorexic or bulimic in pursuit of an unhealthy kind of thinness, keeping weight in the ideal range for your body size is important. It is a basic element of good health.

Did you know that fat cells make estrogen? The fatter you are, the more estrogen your body can make. It also means that all the symptoms of excess estrogen—including having tender breasts before your menstrual period—can worsen. Your risk of cancers that are sensitive to estrogen (breast, ovarian, and uterine [endometrial]) increases. An interesting paradox is that even though an obese woman's body makes more estrogen, she does *not* experience better heart health or heart protection from her obesity. (But the extra estrogen does decrease the risk of osteoporosis—see below.) As discussed in chapter 3, obesity directly threatens heart health and is a major contributor to heart disease—high blood pressure in particular—as the body has to create more blood vessels to get blood to all the excess fat. The extra estrogen produced is not a help here.

In general, African Americans are at low risk for osteoporosis because persons of African heritage have denser skeletal frames. Yet extra estrogen can benefit African American women as far as osteoporosis goes. However, that benefit must be weighed against the increased risk for breast, ovarian, and uterine cancer, along with the increased risk for heart disease caused by obesity, especially from the associated high blood pressure. The presence of sufficient amounts of estrogen helps maintain healthy bones by promoting the storage of calcium, boron, and other necessary minerals in the matrix of bones, keeping them strong. Eating too much protein causes minerals to be taken out of the bones, while eating too little protein makes it difficult for the body to repair tissues made of mostly amino acids, which are the building blocks of protein. Increased force on bones through either weight-bearing exercise (exercise that you perform standing) or purposeful movement of the long bones (arms and legs) also stimulates the storage of calcium and other minerals into the bones. So a combination of hormonal, nutritional influences, and exercise levels contribute to the overall health, density, and strength of your bones. However, there is a balance point with respect to how your body responds to increased weight on the bones. If you are in the healthful range of weight, your bones get the stimulation they need to stay strong when you exercise. In this range, the bones and the joints that connect them are not overwhelmed and normal function remains possible. While someone who weighs too much may not have high risk for osteoporosis, carrying around the excess weight puts too much strain on their joints and can be a source of pain and decreased mobility, making it harder to exercise and help burn off the excess fat.

If what I've said sounds like a contradiction, step back for a moment and reread the previous sentences. Then consider this situation again. If you are obese, your body can produce more estrogen than it needs. While this excess can theoretically provide protection against the problems that can occur when a woman's body does not have enough estrogen—osteoporosis—the excess estrogen a fatter body makes provides no protection against heart disease. The benefit only applies to osteoporosis, a condition for which you are at low risk anyway. Not much benefit comes from the extra weight. Please don't read this as permission to hang on to your extra weight. If you've read chapter 3, you know how much harder your heart has to work to carry it around. When considering estrogen issues, losing the unnecessary weight is the smartest way to go. That extra weight wears out joints, gives your heart more work to do, and increases the risk for a variety of cancers that are estrogen sensitive. These side effects and risks simply cannot justify any supposed benefits from additional estrogen that your body can produce above what it needs and can use.

If you are obese or simply overweight, the best thing you can do for your overall health is to take off the unneeded weight safely and gradually over time. Avoid fad diets and starvation plans like the plague; they do not work over the long haul. Estrogen replacement therapy may be safe and appropriate for you if you have no family history of cancer, especially cancer of the uterus, ovaries, or breast, are at high risk for osteoporosis or heart disease, and your fat cells are not making lots of excess estrogen. Strive to get the lowest possible dose of estrogen to give you the benefits you seek and at the same time minimize your risk of possible serious side effects. Discuss with your doctor whether it makes sense to add progesterone to your dose of estrogen, to take progesterone alone, or to take nothing at all.

It's your body, and you have to live with the decisions you and your health care practitioner make. Be sure to do your part by doing your homework; get information from a variety of sources and weigh all your options. Do your own thinking so you understand exactly what it is you are choosing and the consequences of these choices. In the Resources section of the appendix, I list some other books you may find helpful.

Corticosteroids

I add this section for women who use steroids such as cortisone for whatever reason. Corticosteroids are prescription drugs that are used for their strong anti-inflammatory effects. They are typically prescribed in situations where inflammation can cause major problems, such as significant acute physical trauma, asthma, severe allergies, lupus, and arthritis. Long-term use of corticosteroids is known to cause osteoporosis. If you take these drugs, you should consult with your doctor and do your own reading on this topic, as each situation is individual. Whether ERT is appropriate for you revolves around the balance between your risk for osteoporosis; heart disease; and cancers of the breast, ovaries, or uterus; and whether you are currently obese. Your family history is a factor here, as are all the elements of your lifestyle and environmental exposures. Do you have a family history of cancer among female blood relatives on your mother's side? Make sure your doctor has this important information and that you understand its significance.

Estrogen: Synthetic or Natural?

Before you decide whether synthetic or natural ERT is for you—if that's what you and your health care provider decide is best—it's important that you know more about estrogen.

Did you know that there are three kinds of estrogen? Their names are estrone, estradiol, and estriol. An easy way to remember them is to look at the letters at the end of the word and it tells you which one it is. Estrone (one) is E1, estradiol (di-two) is E2, and estriol (tri-three) is E3. From the beginning of puberty until menopause, these three estrogens appear in a woman's body in the ratio of E1:E2:E3 as 1:1:8. Currently, estradiol is thought to be the friendliest of the three by producing the most benefits and fewest side effects.

Debate continues over whether natural estrogen and synthetic estrogen differ in effectiveness. Currently available on the market and most commonly used are estrogens derived from the soy plant and the urine of pregnant female horses (mares). For many years, Premarin (**pregnant mare urine**) was the most prescribed drug in the United States. Now there are concerns that it may cause more harm than good, and it should only be used by women at high risk for osteoporosis and, perhaps, heart disease, if they do not have significant risk for cancers of the breast, uterus, or ovaries.

Are plant-based estrogens really more friendly, or do many women simply feel better about them because the source is a plant and not the urine harvested from a penned-up pregnant horse? In my clinical experience, most women seem to tolerate plant-based estrogens better than synthetic ones, reporting fewer or no side effects compared with synthetic estrogen. If the estrogen was prescribed to get the woman through menopausal difficulties, then she can gradually wean herself readily when the menopausal changes are finished. Studies have shown that most women stop taking estrogen within three to five years of it being prescribed and taper the doses to ease themselves off of it.

Estrogen taken by mouth has whole-body (systemic) effects. When estrogen is applied as a vaginal cream, it can provide the missing vaginal lubrication needed for more comfortable sexual intercourse. Many women experience a dry, irritated vagina after menopause, even when there was enough foreplay and stimulation for sexual arousal and lubrication. That is, what might have been sufficient foreplay to achieve lubrication for intercourse before menopause isn't effective after menopause without supplementing additional lubrication because the lowered amount of estrogen after menopause leaves the vaginal tissue drier and thinner.

Osteoporosis

Do Black women have the same risk of osteoporosis as women of other races and ethnicities? This is a very interesting question. And what does osteoporosis have to do with heart disease? Directly, not a lot. Indirectly, it can be used as a marker for estrogen status, as it protects bone health in women and heart health in some women.

It was my observation as a child that very elderly Black women in my community seemed to walk straighter than their White counterparts. This observation held both for the extremely petite women and the tall, broadly built women. I did not know the name for what I observed until I became an adult and heard about osteoporosis. From my childhood memories, I thought it looked like not all elderly women and men were evenly affected by this symptom. Admittedly, these were casual observations by a child growing up in Philadelphia, Pennsylvania, and not part of a controlled study. Yet to the untrained eye, it was apparent that there might be something different going on, a phenomenon that was yet unknown to me but clearly at work in the differences in the humped-back (also called "dowager's hump") appearance of these people afflicted with grossly apparent osteoporosis.

It is striking that given today's knowledge of risk factors for osteoporosis, Americans' logic about this illness and how to treat it is lacking. The people most at risk for osteoporosis are women of all races with petite bony frames, especially White women; added factors are long-term low estrogen levels and lack of exercise, especially weight-bearing exercise, that moves the long bones (arms and legs) of the body. White women have the biggest risk for osteoporosis, and yet this same group also consumes the most dairy products as part of its cultural tradition. If milk really does do a body good and contains easily absorbed calcium in plentiful amounts, then why do White women have the highest risk of osteoporosis?

African and Asian cuisines provide calcium in the form of leafy green vegetables, such as collards, mustard greens, kale, and bok choi; seeds such as sesame seeds; sesame seed butter, or tahini; and seafood, such as salmon and sardines. Osteoporosis risk is not as high in these groups of women. Could it be that these vegetable, seed, and seafood sources of calcium are more effectively used by the body in creating healthy hearts, bones, and nervous systems?

People of African heritage are primarily blood type O. Blood type O is the original human blood type; blood types A, B, and AB came later. Blood type O people of any race or ethnicity are least able to digest milk as adults. They lack the enzyme called "lactase" that digests the milk sugar called "lactose." Or, on the other hand, maybe it's that a fraction of the smaller group of people with types A, B, and AB blood just have excess lactase. It's all in how you look at it. Typically in the world of science, if a majority of a population of any kind experiences a phenomenon, then that phenomenon is used as the reference point against which similar phenomena are measured. Oddly, in this case, the tables are turned. Given that 85 percent of the world's population does not digest milk as adults, it is strange that this vast majority is labeled as being deficient in the lactase enzyme.

Perhaps adults were never intended to consume milk of any kind, except for emergencies. Mother's milk is a perfect food for very young humans but is not adequate for adult humans. Maybe it is time to reframe this discussion of milk on the national level from the point of view of a small percentage, about 15 percent, of the world's population that can digest milk into adulthood as that group experiencing lactase *excess* rather than label everyone else as *deficient*. This is definitely something to think about.

A Special Note about Milk and Dairy

For the sake of clarity, it is important to know that "dairy" is defined as products derived from milk such as butter, cream, yogurt, cheese, and cream cheese. Dairy products do not include eggs, which is a common misunderstanding.

Does milk really do a body good? Milk—cow's milk—is rather alkaline, and therefore the minerals in it are not very bioavailable (readily absorbed). Minerals, including calcium, are best absorbed through the stomach, which is normally acidic. This means that the average adult cannot digest the minerals found in cow's milk (such as calcium) very well. Milk is also a mucous-forming food and is considered damp and congesting from an Eastern medicine point of view.

Most of the world's people cannot digest and assimilate milk as adults. In fact, after the age of three or four years, about 85 percent of the world's population loses the ability to properly digest milk from mammals, especially cows. Some people seem to better tolerate goat's milk or sheep's milk and cheeses made from these milks. The human gut best digests human mother's milk when we are babies and toddlers.

The human digestive tract and immune system react normally to mother's milk. Milk from animals of other species are less tolerated by infants and toddlers, and cow's milk is tolerated least. In some children, cow's milk causes repeated ear infections, colds, asthma, sinusitis, and chronic excess excretion of mucous from the child's throat, nose, and eyes.

Do you experience uncomfortable symptoms after eating dairy products? Gas, abdominal bloating or pain, burping, nausea, diarrhea, alternating diarrhea and constipation, foul-smelling stools, coughing up mucous, feeling a constant need to clear the throat, mucous at the corners of the eyes, unexplained rashes, eczema, asthma, allergies, and other food or environmental sensitivities are the most common cluster of symptoms that indicate a person may have a problem with digesting milk products. Are any of these symptoms familiar? Some symptoms can be delayed up to four days. Recognizing these symptoms depends on how reactive your body is to milk and related substances, as well as how many other background health problems exist that may make it difficult to recognize the symptoms of lactose intolerance.

Some patients experience significant weight loss after they stop eating dairy products, especially milk, cheese, and ice cream. The weight loss remains for as long as they remove dairy products from their diet. This result was consistent no matter whether the person drank whole milk, skim milk, or other forms of fat-reduced dairy products. Was the weight loss due to increased metabolism or a loss of the excess mucous caused by milk consumption? Was weight loss caused by better performance of the person's insulin and its ability to use glucose (blood sugar)? Or was it caused by a shift in the metabolism towards burning fat rather than storing it? These are all interesting questions to explore.

Other patients report that their chronic sinus congestion clears up and remains gone provided they stay off of dairy products. Similarly, many patients report that their allergy symptoms lessen and asthma attacks are less frequent and less severe when they're not consuming dairy.

We know that people of African and Asian heritage are least able to digest dairy products as adults. It is interesting to note that the foods traditionally eaten for centuries by these cultures do not contain dairy products in large amounts. In fact, many of the cuisines of these cultures do not contain dairy products at all, yet osteoporosis rates among people of African heritage are low.

Dairy and Babies

If you think about it, milk is really for the young of a species. This means that human milk is for baby humans, sheep's milk is for baby sheep, and cow's milk is for baby cows. Ironically, friends from rural areas have told me that even baby cows do not drink cow's milk. What do they know that we don't?

Research has shown that cow's milk causes type I (childhood-onset) diabetes in some children, as their immune system is triggered to attack their own pancreas, the specific place where insulin is made. The cells in the islets of Langerhans in the pancreas are where the damage is done, and the body then no longer makes its own insulin; this creates a requirement for insulin from outside the body, either taken by mouth (oral) or by injection. What a price to pay for drinking milk. It isn't known yet who is at risk for this reaction.

Today there are nondairy options for baby formulas, some of which are soy based. Some children are sensitive or truly allergic to soy products. This becomes an issue if you use a soy-based infant formula. Check with your health professional about feeding options if you are not breastfeeding, as most soy milk, almond milk, rice milk, and oat milk products that are not specifically labeled as infant formulas are not a substitute for more wholesome baby formulas. These other milks do not contain the right balance of amino acids (a kind of protein), essential fatty acids, and vitamins to give the rapidly developing baby enough nourishment. The nutritional needs of infants are not the same as those of teenagers, adults, or elders. Some of the most common commercial brands of infant formulas have lots of sugar, artificial ingredients, and other items that may not directly contribute to the optimal health of the baby. Read labels carefully and ask questions of qualified persons if you have any doubts about this.

We all have to make our own choices about dairy products, but you may want to consider saying good-bye to dairy. For many of us, it makes the most sense. But that doesn't mean we don't need calcium. Calcium remains an important mineral for all women. Not only is it important to get as much calcium as possible from calcium-rich foods like leafy greens (cooked healthily, of course), but it may be important for you to take calcium as a supplement. The soils that foods are grown in today are depleted of vital nutrients, including minerals.

Put It All Together

Cow's milk is not a good source of needed minerals like calcium. Calcium is required along with boron, manganese, and vitamin D for healthy bones. Exercise that moves the long bones of the body is also required for healthy bones. These same factors also contribute to healthy hearts.

We don't live our lives in test tubes. The scientific model of the world is limited by what it can teach us that we need to know about the factors that influence health. In a controlled study environment, it is possible to look at one factor at a time in relative isolation and observe its influence on the final result of an experiment. This test tube oriented study method has value, and there is definitely a place for this approach and the information it brings. Balance between common sense and scientific findings is needed to really maximize the help these two approaches can offer. There is definitely a need for both. One in the absence of the other is not an optimal approach.

American Heart Association, *1999 Heart and Stroke Statistical Update*, (Dallas, Texas: American Heart Association 1999),11.

Chapter 9
Black Women and Smoking

It's best to never start smoking, and if you do smoke, quit now. The good news: In the United States, Black women as a group have the lowest rates of people taking up smoking for the first time.

The bad news: For Black women who do smoke, the negative impact of smoking is out of proportion to the number of cigarettes and other tobacco products smoked or otherwise consumed. Black women get sick more easily and intensely from the effects of tobacco smoke, nicotine, and related chemical byproducts such as cotinine, a derivative of nicotine.

I've considered all of the reasons people smoke and the reasons why people quit smoking, and I think it is important to keep the big picture of actions and consequences in perspective. The discussions I've had over the years both with people who smoke and people who have quit smoking have provided great information and poignant contrast about the values people have about smoking.

I have noticed that those who successfully quit smoking, always win the mental and spiritual battle first. Their minds are made up that they will quit no matter how hard it gets, and they do indeed quit. These people are also less likely to have a really difficult time quitting, as they usually do not give themselves any built-in excuses or backup plans "just in case" their plans to quit fail. It may take more than one attempt to quit smoking, but quit they do. Given nicotine's powerful chemical addiction, this is a strong acknowledgment of the power of mind over matter.

If you are going to quit smoking, do everything you can to stack the odds in your favor. Be fully committed to ending a habit that has absolutely no benefits and many risks for you. You and your health are worth the challenge of quitting—for good.

Ten Good Reasons to Smoke

The following list identifies the possible results of smoking. It is intended as a wake-up call for readers who are unaware of how this habit ruins health and worsens diseases and illness. It is not meant to be a mockery, simply a plainly worded, "tell it like it is" list of possibilities associated with smoking.

- You want to die early.
- You want to greatly increase your chances of dying of lung cancer.
- You want to increase your chances of dying of other kinds of cancer, emphysema, or other lung and breathing disorders.
- You want your clothes and breath to smell bad to most people.
- You want your teeth to have yellow stains.
- You do not want to taste food and smell odors at your full potential.
- You can't figure out what else to do during break time at work.
- It's the cheapest, easiest way you can figure out to soothe your frazzled nerves that's legal.
- Smoking keeps you from gaining weight. Every time you quit, here come the pounds.
- You feel powerless over this addiction.

Ten Good Reasons to Smoke

There isn't even so much as one good reason to smoke, never mind 10 good reasons. Just wanted to see if you were paying attention. But for fun, let's review a list anyway.

Do these comments seem harsh? They are. So is what smoking does to your body. You deserve better.

Some good news: There is help available. For people who want to stop smoking, some of the most effective natural treatments include acupuncture; herbal combinations taken as teas, tinctures, or supplements; prayer; and biofeedback.

"Well, I'm gonna die anyway of somethin', so it might as well be this . . . . "

Research and common sense are proving that quality of life often determines quantity of life for most people. So if we never take care of ourselves, constantly burn the candle at both ends, and have little life enjoyment, it is likely that we will die earlier than average, and dying is more likely to be a painful, harsh experience as well.

Smoking causes its own set of illnesses, like emphysema, lung cancer, asthma, pneumonia, and chronic bronchitis. It also worsens just about every other illness, especially heart disease. Smoking is the one contributing factor to heart disease that is the most preventable. Never smoke. It's as simple as that.

For Black women, there are issues tied up with smoking, just as there are for any group of people. Consider the incredible sorrows and ongoing injustices our ancestors had to bear, the heartbreak and tragedies unique to Black slave women. Remember that there is no reason to ever doubt our ability to do anything; this includes giving up cigarettes forever.

In terms of our collective history, stopping smoking has to be easier than escaping from a plantation or being tortured in pursuit of freedom, and it has to be easier than getting the right to vote in the United States. If need be, lean on the strength, faith, and perseverance of our ancestors to get you through any tough spots you encounter when letting cigarettes and other tobacco products go for good. Those cigarettes don't have anything to offer you that is truly in your best interests.

Business Aspects of Smoking

As the market for tobacco products shrinks in the United States, manufacturers scramble to develop new markets in other parts of the world so they can maintain or increase their sales and revenue growth. The ranks of U.S. smokers are steadily decreasing, in part because many people quit smoking, current smokers are dying off, and fewer people take up the habit.

This interest in developing new markets is normal for any business, especially an international business. The problem for the tobacco industry is that their products can wreak havoc on customers' health. Many people feel that for this reason these kinds of products should be banned or at least limited in their availability. In the United States, sales of tobacco products are restricted by age and the products are heavily taxed. These factors, along with the increasing cost of the product, the social stigma associated with smoking, and the reality of the diseases caused by smoking, have combined to help decrease the overall rate of smoking in the United States.

Recent investigations have proven that tobacco products have been engineered to give a consistent delivery of nicotine, a key chemical in the tobacco addiction process. Because of this deliberate manipulation of tobacco's chemical content and its effects on the body of the smoker, smokers have a consistent "good" experience when they smoke. Remember that smoking is a choice people make. No matter how seductive or skilled the marketing tactics are, each one of us has the choice to smoke or not smoke. Keep in mind that it's a choice.

I remember the first time I was introduced to the possibility that tobacco products were altered, processed, or genetically engineered in a way that made them more addictive and more physically harmful. I was in my second year of naturopathic medical school in the early 1990s when our pathology professor commented that the rates of disease and illness associated with smokers were not uniform around the world. He stated that the highest rates of disease and illness seemed to occur wherever tobacco products that were made in the United States were sold. He also commented that smokers in other countries usually smoked fewer cigarettes per person than U.S. smokers; chain-smoking was not typical in these other societies. Our professor said that there was speculation that U.S.-manufactured tobacco was altered in some way that might account for the differences in the addiction, disease, and illness rates associated with smoking around the world.

For many years, there were denials about whether tobacco was altered or processed in a way that changed its inherent chemistry or how smoking interacted with human biochemistry. Now that investigators have discovered the extent to which tobacco products are processed and altered, smokers are realizing that they have been set up to be even more deeply addicted to a product that was quite addictive on its own in its original form. Because smoking is addictive, attempts by the manufacturers of tobacco to "standardize" their product have had extraordinary impact on and implications for the health consequences of smoking.

Social Aspects of Smoking

Whatever social bonding may occur between smokers as they huddle outside buildings to smoke simply isn't worth the risk. Some smokers, especially women, feel that their cigarettes are always there for them, like a kind of friend that is constantly available. This is a misplaced feeling. Among my female patients who smoke or used to smoke, this is the most common reason they smoke.

It's much better to develop real friends, actual people you can talk to and count on as buddies and confidantes, than to leave that personal connection unfulfilled, empty of people who recognize how special you are and can act on it in positive ways. Sucking on a lit piece of paper filled with dried shredded leaves and inhaling the smoke is no substitute for fulfilling friendships and caring people in your life. Accept no substitutes for genuine, loving relationships. Grow and nurture connections with positive, caring, and reliable people.

Recently I've had some conversations with women who are what I call "casual" smokers; they smoke a couple of times a month and claim they are not addicted to cigarettes. The reasons these people give for smoking on occasion are that it helps them to feel more "grounded" or that they feel "closer" to certain people in their lives who are dead now, kind of like communing with the spirits. As I was running one morning, I realized what was funny (peculiar) about their comments. Maybe these people really were trying to be "closer" and "grounded" through smoking; smoking would bring them closer to being in the ground—in a coffin! Hmmm. Something to think about.

"My nerves are bad . . . . "

What an interesting expression. This phrase is the most common refrain I have heard from African American women over the years as the number one reason they smoke. These smokers say that smoking calms them, soothes jangled nerves, and helps them to feel like they can respond to anything. They also say that the act of smoking gives them time to think. You know, it's peculiar. Athletes say similar things about running and other kinds of exercise. People who meditate regularly talk about the quieting and soothing effect meditation has on their soul and psyche. Yet these athletic and meditative activities do not inflict damage like smoking does. It's interesting that such different behaviors can be associated with the same feelings and experiences that people seek. Whatever the reasons given for smoking, it is hard to ever find a way to justify it as a sensible activity.

From a technical point of view, there is no such thing as "bad nerves." If this is some of the self-talk you have about smoking, recognize it for what it is: a story you tell yourself to excuse the fact you lean on cigarettes like a crutch. Face it. Your nerves are not really bad. You may simply lack the skills that help you find other ways to deal with stress. Facing the truth of this situation can set you free to make needed changes. Lying to yourself keeps you trapped. No significant change can happen as long as these internal lies keep you hypnotized and blinded against your own real power to stop smoking for good.

I think it's time we hold ourselves to a new standard of health and take full accountability for the state of our health. There are people today who are on respirators or who have emphysema due to the damage smoking did to their lungs, wheezing with every breath in a desperate attempt to get enough air in so that they can breathe. Consider that the average person takes a breath six times a minute. Imagine struggling day after day simply to breathe. When smoking became very popular and fashionable in the 1940s and 1950s, the long-term effects of smoking were not well known. Today there is no such excuse, as the consequences of smoking are well established.

We have the most to gain from positive changes. Our health destiny is in our hands; we determine our destiny by the choices we make every day. I do not want to hold back at all on this topic and leave any reader with the impression that there is anything OK about smoking. There simply is nothing good to be said about it.

Do I make myself clear?

The Impact of Smoking

OK, why is smoking such a big darn deal, especially as it relates to heart health? The nicotine in inhaled smoke from tobacco and related smoking products directly damages the walls of blood vessels. This is corrosion from the inside out, and it contributes to risk that fats in the blood will stick to the walls of the blood vessel and cause blockages that are called atherosclerosis. This increases the risk of clots that can turn into embolisms (clots on the move) that travel via the bloodstream and get stuck in other blood vessels, such as the coronary arteries in the heart (causing a heart attack), in the brain (causing a stroke), or in the lungs (causing a pulmonary embolism).

In addition to creating a chemical addiction, nicotine is also a potent constrictor of blood vessels. It causes the blood vessel to significantly narrow. This means that less blood flows through the blood vessel under higher pressure, causing the heart to work harder and harder delivering blood to the tissues that it serves.

The impact of smoking does not stop with the heart. Smoking impacts the body in the following ways:
- raises blood pressure
- damages blood vessels
- worsens atherosclerosis, the buildup of fat in blood vessel linings
- adds to blood congestion by speeding up clot formation
- causes or worsens sinusitis
- causes lung cancer

- causes mouth cancer
- causes other kinds of cancer
- causes emphysema, bronchitis, pneumonia, asthma
- causes mouth ulcers
- during pregnancy:
  increases risk of miscarriage
  increases risk of premature delivery
  increases risk of low birth weight of infant
  increases risk of sudden infant death syndrome (SIDS)

All of these factors, separately and in combination, are potent forces that greatly increase the risk of heart attacks, strokes, embolisms, high blood pressure, and other forms of heart disease. These increased risks of serious illness are quite a price to pay for the temporary pleasure or distraction that smoking offers. It simply isn't worth the trouble it causes.

To give you a reference for the addictive power of nicotine, it's considered to be somewhere from 10 to 100 times more addictive than morphine or its common derivative, heroin. While it's difficult to quit smoking, millions of people can attest to the fact that it *is* possible to permanently stop smoking. It takes commitment, discipline, and a focus on the results that accompany the cessation of smoking. It's definitely worth the work involved.

Smoking takes a terrible toll on the body and on the health of the smoker. (And, as we now know, smoking also takes a toll on the health of the people around the smoker, those who must inhale secondhand smoke.) But what happens, you may ask, if you stop smoking?

Our bodies have an amazing capacity to recover when we stop smoking. Particularly remarkable is the ability of the lung tissue to initiate and sustain repairs to damaged respiratory tissues. The lungs have a very large surface area for the exchange of oxygen and carbon dioxide, and much of the long-term repair occurs there.

Some interesting and very positive changes occur after someone stops smoking. Twenty minutes after smoking their last cigarette, the smoker's blood pressure returns to normal or significantly decreases. The smoker's risk of having a heart attack decreases 24 hours after the last cigarette is consumed. The benefits continue over time. Over the next month to one year, a new nonsmoker experiences decreased sinus congestion, decreased shortness of breath, and decreased coughing as the lungs start to clear themselves of the damage and chemical residue (tar and nicotine byproducts) that was deposited with each cigarette smoked. After 10 years of being smoke-free, the ex-smoker has half the risk for lung cancer they had while they smoked.

Black Folks and Smoking

Recent studies have shown that African Americans may be more vulnerable than other racial and ethnic groups to the harmful side effects of smoking. The reason appears to be that a key element of the addictive and disease-causing chemical nicotine called cotinine (a byproduct of nicotine made by the person's body) stays in the blood of Black smokers longer than in White, Hispanic, or Asian smokers. The studies showed that this higher level of cotinine in the blood of Black smokers was found no matter how many cigarettes per day were smoked. This means that the chemicals of smoke have a longer time to circulate in the blood and potentially do damage to the lungs, heart, blood vessels, and so on. At this time, it is not known why Black smokers have higher levels of cotinine in the blood after smoking.

Blood levels of cotinine (nicotine derivative) for African Americans:
12%–50% higher than those in Whites
32%–56% higher than those in Mexican Americans

Research has shown that African Americans who smoke are at higher risk than Whites of developing lung cancer and dying from it. These research results may help explain the higher rate of death due to lung cancer among Black smokers compared to White smokers. Other research has shown that Black smokers tend to smoke fewer cigarettes than White smokers, inhale more deeply while smoking, and hold the smoke in their lungs for a longer period of time. The relative popularity of menthol cigarettes among Black smokers may further compound the problem, as the anaesthetizing effect of menthol could mean that a smoker will inhale mentholated smoke more deeply into their lungs, increasing the contact time with lung tissue and the amount of lung tissue directly exposed to the smoke. These facts make it even more important to quit if you do smoke, and to never begin if you do not smoke.

Studies also show that Blacks are more likely than other groups of people to try to quit smoking, to try more frequently to quit smoking, and to have more difficulty actually quitting smoking. (However, once they quit, Blacks are also more likely to never resume smoking again.) This difference in the success rate of quitting smoking may be explained by the higher levels of cotinine, which suggest that Blacks absorb more nicotine from cigarettes than do other groups.

All of these research results mean that it may be harder for African American smokers to quit, as they experience the double whammy of deeper pleasure and a deeper addiction from the chemicals in cigarettes. It doesn't mean that quitting is impossible. It just acknowledges that the degree of difficulty may be different, so do everything you can to put the odds in your favor. Keep this possibility in mind and use it to your advantage to celebrate in healthy ways as you begin and finish the path to quitting smoking. A positive attitude and absolute commitment to stopping smoking for good are essential to your success.

Advertising Trends for Smoking

As previously mentioned, tobacco products companies tailor their business practices to maximize sales of their products. When these products have significant negative health impacts, these tactics become problematic.

Successful businesses conduct extensive market research so the company gets the most exposure and revenue possible from all market segments served. For some products, marketing and advertising campaigns target all parts of the population, while others focus on what the company perceives to be either its "mainstream" or core audience—the audience on which it has the most influence and from which it gets the biggest return for the money it invests in promotional activities. For years, Blacks and other U.S. minorities felt left out or underrepresented in advertising for many products. As various companies responded, there was a shift in advertising that resulted in an increase in the ads targeted to racial and ethnic audiences.

Since White smokers were quitting smoking more easily and at a faster rate than Black smokers, tobacco products companies increased their efforts to grow their market share in racial and ethnic communities, including Black communities. Different brands of cigarettes were advertised in different communities. The whole concept of brand development dictates that advertising programs target consumers specifically so that they can recognize that the product is for them; then, with this recognition, consumers will buy it over and over again. So goes the theory of brand development and recognition. Menthol cigarette billboard ads were most common in Black neighborhoods, and these ads appeared in magazines targeted at Black consumers. Old West or Wild West (United States) and cowboy theme cigarettes ads were most common in White neighborhoods, especially lower-income White neighborhoods.

Given the health consequences of smoking, this targeted advertising had a larger negative impact in the community in terms of the results in real people's lives. Years later, restrictions were placed on the promotion and advertising of tobacco products in an effort to slow the rise of disease and illness associated with smoking and other forms of tobacco product consumption.

Despite the restrictions placed on the promotion and advertising of tobacco products, tobacco companies still market their wares and make them attractive to the consumer. It is interesting to observe the current increased popularity of cigar smoking and where the advertising for cigars is placed, given that cigars have been typically associated with success, celebrations, and affluence. Cigars deliver three to four times the nicotine per inhalation than cigarettes do, giving the smoker even more of a rush as they smoke the cigar. Cigars' association with celebrities increases the perception in the minds of potential smokers that this is an OK thing to do; after all, Famous Person _____ does it, so it can't be all bad. This classic use of manipulative advertising does not serve anyone in the pursuit of better health and wellness.

Specific Smoking Risks for Black Women

For Black women, the risks to heart health from smoking are high. Why, you ask? I'll tell you. Consider that when most people are stressed, they'll do

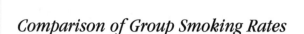

Comparison of Group Smoking Rates

For Black women, there is a positive note here: compared to Black men, White women, and White men, Black women have the lowest rate of people taking up smoking for the first time. This is important, as people who never start smoking avoid all of the problems associated with it. Let us as a community do all we can to drive this number even lower and encourage others to join us in never beginning to smoke.

Percentage of group who smokes:

African American women	22.7%	White women	24.4%
African American men	31%	White men	28%

In the past, Black adults smoked at higher rates than the general population. In recent years, this has shifted as Black adults have smoked at about the same rates as other groups. In the mid-1970s, smoking rates among Black teenagers dropped dramatically; recently, the rate has begun to climb again. If you know any teens who smoke, be sure to share this chapter with them.

anything to relieve the stress. Consider also that when people are stressed, they are most likely to do what is easiest to get rid of stress. For the average person in a typical situation, it is easier to smoke than it is to do health-promoting things, like exercise or meditate, as a way to deal with the feelings of stress. Stress affects all human beings to some degree. Our ability to cope with stress in healthful ways will determine the short-term and long-term consequences that stress will have on our lives.

Many Black women have increased amounts of stress due to the following:
• more likely to have low income (financial stress),
• higher debts (A black woman may be charged more for the same item

than someone who is not Black, not female, or both. Example: research has demonstrated that Black women pay more for cars than any other group of people after adjustments for income, credit worthiness, and negotiating skills.)
- lack of access to better financing terms or ignorance of financial options
- jobs that don't allow for independent action or expression
- racism
- sexism
- long-term unemployment or underemployment
- have more young children and no mate to raise them with
- experiencing the "sandwich phenomenon" (In this situation, the woman tends two generations in her family or extended family: the children she is raising and the elders she is caring for. In some families, the "sandwich phenomenon" shifts to the elder members: the grandmother tends to the grandchildren she is raising and the elders she is caring for. This woman may find herself raising her grandchildren because the children she raised are not caring for their own children, as one might expect.)

This increased exposure to social stresses nudge (maybe shove) Black women toward compensating for the extra stress with quick fixes like smoking. (It appears that smoking is an acquired habit;, no genetic or inherited risk for smoking has been discovered as it has for alcoholism.) For Black women, internalizing feelings of stress can become an emotional powder keg, and the "blowup" usually occurs at the expense of their health. Avoid keeping feelings in. Express them in useful ways so they don't build up over time only to make you sick seemingly out of the blue years later.

As I mentioned earlier, smoking causes heart disease by narrowing the blood vessels and damaging the side walls of blood vessels. This contributes to increased speed of blood clotting, high blood pressure, and atherosclerosis (the build up of fatty plaques on the walls of blood vessels); all of these together greatly increase the risk of heart attacks, strokes, and worsening of other kinds of heart disease. Smoking causes other direct damage, such as sinusitis and lung cancer. Smoking during pregnancy harms the baby, increasing the risk of miscarriage, premature delivery, low birth weight, and sudden infant death syndrome. Our smoking, then, is not only bad for us; it is bad for those we love as well.

What about other people around those who smoke? Smoking affects nonsmokers through secondhand smoke. Nonsmokers exposed to cigarette smoke have increased rates of lung disease, heart disease, and cancer. Smoke is powerful in its effects for both people who smoke and those around them who don't. If for some reason people who smoke cannot quit, then they should take every precaution to avoid exposing the people around them to smoke. There is no point in spreading the health damage and disease risks around.

Precautions concerning exposure to smoke especially apply to children. Unlike adult nonsmokers, they are not as able to do anything about their exposure to smoke. For example, smoking in the car with the windows cracked "for fresh air" is not good enough. Changes in the wind and other factors often cause the smoke to blow back into the car, affecting everyone in it.

By smoking—or hopefully, by not smoking—adults set an example for children. Children watch what their parents and other relatives do; which is even more important than what they say to the children. If children hear the adults in their lives say, "Never mind what I do; do what I say," and yet the children continually witness hypocrisy, they are likely to imitate the adults out of curiosity; they will want to find out about the appeal of such activities. Children who grow up around adults who smoke are more likely to at least try smoking, since they look up to the adults around them and figure that if the adults do it, it must be OK in some way. After all, the adults wouldn't really do something that was clearly bad for them, would they?

The best way for adults to make it clear to children that smoking is not a good thing is to not smoke. Consistency goes a long way in teaching young people the value of anything, including taking care of one's health. Be sure to give yourself and your children consistent healthful messages. You'll be glad you did, now and in the future.

Strategies for Black Women Concerning Smoking

Take responsibility for what you associate with smoking—whether it's pleasure, rebellion, distraction, something you feel you can count on, con-

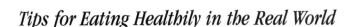

Tips for Eating Healthily in the Real World

Job Stress

Many people turn to foods for comfort when they feel stressed. The way to work off stress is to exercise, exercise, exercise. This lets your body burn up the chemicals it makes as a response to stress and blow off the sensations that often accompany stress, such as chronically tight shoulders and shallow breathing patterns. The chemicals that are released as part of an appropriate stress response can do quite a bit of harm floating around in your bloodstream; their chronic presence damages your body. It is far better for you to work it off than to let it hang around too long and cause harm to your blood vessels.

Reach only for healthy snacks. No cheating with junky foods under the guise of "you deserve a treat." The real treat is treating yourself well by taking care of yourself in a consistent fashion. But if you blow it and go back to less healthy habits, don't beat yourself up about it. Acknowledge the mistake and write down why you got off track. Promise yourself that you'll do better next time on behalf of your health.

nection with others who smoke, or simply a way to pass the time. As long as you take charge of what it means in your own mind and feelings, you can win the battle for your mind and money when it comes to this and any other addictive substance that is so harmful to health.

You must always look out for your own best interests; this is your job and no one else's. Others are not likely to do this for you, as that may not be in their best interests and may represent an odd kind of caretaking or patronization.

Be your own best friend when it comes to your health and the health of your loved ones. Render yourself immune to attempts to harm, poison, or otherwise decrease the quality and quantity of life that you can enjoy. It is worth the vigilance; the payback continues over the course of your lifetime.

Chapter 10
The Mind-Body Connection

As we near the end of this book, we come not to a close but to a beginning (or hopefully a continuation!): you taking excellent care of yourself in all areas of your life. What motivates you to reach for the best possible health, especially heart health? What's the point of all this work?

The purpose of this book is to make available to you all the tools, resources, and inspiration possible to assist you in making life-affirming choices so you can benefit from your own great decisions.

Information is useless without appropriate action. Turn this information into knowledge by making full use of it; raise your expectations of what it means to be well in all areas of your life. Then increase your knowledge and transform it into wisdom by mastering the elements that support heart health.

Make heart healthy habits a part of your daily life and enjoy them. Regardless of your personal circumstances—no matter whether you eat healthy food prepared at home or eat out a lot, whether you're a single parent or you share the parenting role, whether you have lots of job stress or very little, you can make your health a priority and enjoy every day the rich rewards of great health.

Expressions of the Heart

The joyful heart. The glad heart. The heart of courage. A grateful heart. These are a few of the expressions and emotions commonly associated with the heart. Many of the best of human emotions and the most intense emotions are considered to reside in the figurative heart.

We often think of emotions as being more powerful or intense when they are associated with the heart. In your opinion, which sounds more intense and potent: "her mind was filled with rage" or "her heart was brimming with rage"? Compare these two: "her being was infused with a sense of gratitude" versus "her heart overflowed with gratitude, it welled up from deep within her soul, and spilled out to touch everyone who graced her life." Compelling, isn't it? Emotional and provocative associations are tied to descriptions about feelings from the heart.

So let's explore some matters of the heart. What is uplifting to your emotional and spiritual heart? What makes your spirit dance and your soul sing? How important is it to you to have your heart filled with gratitude and joy? Take a few moments now to answer these questions and make a "heart nourishment" list.

Now take a few moments to list those things that "drain" your emotional and spiritual heart. Review what you have listed and the frequency with which these things provide annoyance, irritation, or fatigue. If the list of "heart drainers" is longer or the frequency of draining events is higher than your "heart nourishment" list, look at it as an opportunity for personal growth. If your "heart nourishment" list is significantly longer, congratulations! You are most likely on the right path for creating and maintaining heart health on multiple levels.

To lead a fulfilled life, a life of joy and gratitude with a sense of purpose, you need a balance between the good and the bad, the wanted and the unwanted experiences of life. The human psyche requires contrast, a rich diversity in experiences in order to fully develop and achieve its true potential. For life to be richly and deeply experienced, we all need a variety of events and circumstances that spur our emotional growth and teach our souls the lessons we were born to learn. There are no shortcuts in this process as our souls develop throughout our lifetime. People best acquire confidence and self-esteem through the internal

Expressions of Your Heart

Make a list of the people, places, things, and activities that nourish your emotional heart.

_____   _____

_____   _____

_____   _____

_____   _____

Beside each item you listed, write down how often you have that experience in a month.

Look over what you have listed and the frequency with which these experiences have provided enjoyment, which can also be thought of as "nutrition for the heart and soul." Any insights here for you? Is there room for improvement? Are you feeding your emotional heart in excellent, nurturing ways, or is it getting clogged with toxic waste, junk that you cannot use or that is harmful to you?

Make a list of people, places, things, and activities that drain your emotional heart.

_____   _____

_____   _____

_____   _____

_____   _____

Beside each item you listed, write down how often you have that experience in a month.

Heart Health for Black Women by Dr. Beverly Yates

knowledge that they really can do a particular activity or handle a challenging situation based on their experiences. Whether their choices and responses were effective or ineffective (that is, whether they succeeded or failed) is not the key; what matters is that they got the experience firsthand. What you heard about, read about, or with the best of intentions meant to do are not satisfactory replacements for the real thing, which is getting in there and handling life's surprises as best you can in the moment.

Our beliefs, thoughts, and actions determine our health on all levels, including the physical, mental, emotional, and spiritual realms. Lousy thoughts with great actions are not a good team, and likewise great thoughts with lousy actions are not a good team. Some people think that they can avoid physical exercise by thinking good thoughts, that somehow the power of their mind will compensate for their lack of physical activity—not true! You must have integrity—that is, you must be in congruence, in right alignment with what you want so that your beliefs, thoughts, and actions are in sync with your goals. When this synergy happens, you will be pulled in the direction of what you most desire. It will feel almost effortless, if you remove the inconsistencies that disrupt your integrity. Your personal integrity will shine like a beacon to the other people in your life. You may notice that as your internal and external integrity become completely aligned, you will have more like-minded people in your life. It also will be easier to spot other people's intentions or situations that are not in energetic agreement with the strength and resoluteness of your integrity. This makes life simpler because it gets easier to focus on what you want and eliminate or avoid what you do not want, including people who are heart drainers.

If your life is wonderful now and always has been wonderful, with no major bumps or upsets, good for you! The lack of strife does not make you a lesser person at all. It simply means, without being proactive and seeking out the opportunity to stretch yourself, you haven't directly experienced some things that would require you to stretch beyond your comfort zone. This is quite different from the habit of avoiding challenges and opportunities to grow.

A life that is too easy because you keep ducking growth opportunities, a life history without major problems to solve, is as out of balance as a life in which everything is hard and only gets worse day after day. Sometimes, to develop a grateful heart, you have to look for the good in any given situation, even if the only good thing about it from your perspective is that it is over.

Look at your lists one more time and notice what's good about each of them. Notice where opportunities for improvement lie. Highlight those elements you want to keep or amplify so you have a visual target to focus your efforts on. Circle the elements you want to decrease or eliminate. Write down what you will do, by when you will do it (deadlines are very empowering), and the steps you need to take to make it happen. You have the ability to respond, the "response ability" for making your life go well. The power is in your hands. Use it for your own highest good.

Remove any reason that includes the word "should." Few people ever really take action on the things that they "should" do. They just use these "shoulds" as a way to beat themselves up for failures, both real and imagined. If you can state any reason in a way that eliminates the word "should," then the reason can stay. Example: "I should exercise every day because I know it's good for me" can be rewritten as "I want to exercise every day because I know it will allow me to consistently feel my best." Keep your responses simple and clear. It is much easier to follow simple objectives than to follow grandiose and difficult goals. Clarity about

Three Daily Actions You'll Take to Achieve Great Health

What three specific actions are you willing and able to take each day to create and maintain great health?

_____

_____

_____

My Top 7 Reasons for Great Health

Write down your top seven reasons why you want great health, especially heart health.

_____

_____

_____

_____

_____

_____

_____

what you want gets the job done. It makes it much easier for you to recognize those elements that support your goals and avoid any elements that deter or distract you from attaining your desired results.

Is there anything that keeps you today from taking these three specific actions on behalf of your present and future great health? Use the blank note pages at the back of the book to write down these obstacles (if any), real or perceived.

Now that you've identified these obstacles, review them again while thinking about each one as an opportunity for change. What can you do today—yes, right now—to remove these obstacles? Write down these actions too. This is your record for yourself of how you plan to achieve great health for yourself because you deserve it.

Now take action; follow through and do what you wrote down as action steps to remove obstacles. If it really isn't possible for you to put this book down for a moment and complete all the action steps right this instant, schedule their completion in your daily activities. Most people do what they schedule, so make an appointment with yourself to get this done *now*. I've included the blank note pages in the appendix to give you the opportunity to record your thoughts. Take advantage of this space. It's just for you.

As you've read this book, you may have noticed that I continue to emphasize actions and give you homework to do as we go along. The reason for my focus is that I have repeatedly observed that many people know what to do in their lives, but they don't actually do what they know. Most of us have some idea that exercise and nutrition are our friends for a lifetime of wellness, yet we don't get out of our chairs often enough to get the benefit of our knowledge. Knowing about something useful that can help you is not enough; using that knowledge is what makes the critical difference.

A balance between mental health in the form of quality thought patterns—beliefs that support you in attaining overall health—and actions that get the desired results are an excellent team for you in all the aspects of your life, including the physical, mental, emotional, and spiritual realms. In the purest sense, having the world's best thoughts is an outstanding achievement. Yet these magnificent thoughts require a physical home worthy of them. In other words, you must balance thoughts, feelings, and spiritual activities with the needs of your physical self. Neglecting one realm at the expense of the others is not a good long-term solution. For practical reasons, you may focus on one particular area of your life. Keep in mind that it is important to maintain forward progress in all areas of your life as you go on in your journey.

You may have also noticed as you read along in this book that I continue to ask you to write things down and not just keep them in your head. Why, you ask? In this way, you can maximize the benefit you receive from the exercises included here. Our brains process information that we write differently than they do those things we speak or type in a computer or on a typewriter. There is something about the act of writing that allows knowledge to go deeper and increases the likelihood of remembering the information and then taking appropriate actions on that information. Our nervous system stores that knowledge more easily and then allows us to more readily access it when we need to remember it for current use. As a test, the next time you are in a meeting or another situation where you need to track information, take notes and review them that night. You will see for yourself the difference in your ability to remember the key points from the meeting.

The Heart of Giving

There is something powerful and freeing in regularly giving to others. It makes you feel good on the inside.

Whether you tithe at church or another place of spiritual worship; donate money, services, or goods to charities; or volunteer your time and skills to a worthy cause, you are invoking the power of universal reciprocity. These simple acts invite more of life's goodness into your daily experience. You can make it a habit to give regularly in this fashion and participate in the flow of life. Sharing your offerings with the world helps to leave it a better place than you found it.

Do you give to yourself on a regular basis in a way that is good for you? I mean really good, not superficial. Do you give yourself time for massages, warm baths with aromatherapy essential oils, lunches with your buddies, phone calls to people you love and trust? Are you learning about nutrition and exercise? Do you create enough quiet time around you to notice what is good in your life and what is going well? Do you give yourself credit for the things you have learned and the courage it takes to learn new things in your life? Do you give yourself forgiveness as needed for your shortcomings? Do you give yourself and others enough room in your life to show your own and their imperfections? Do you give in a way that you know will have the best possible impact?

Are you generous? Do you consider yourself a generous person? What does the word "generous" mean to you? How do you show your generosity? Do you expect others to acknowledge your acts of generosity? Why or why not? There are no right or wrong answers to these questions. How you respond determines to some extent how good you feel about yourself on the inside and, consequently, what you show to the world. Ideally your "outer you" will reflect the inner richness that is the real you. If there is a major disharmony between what you feel on the inside and what you show on the outside, well, here's another opportunity for positive change to get the "inner you" and "outer you" in alignment. Energy flows most easily when there are no obstructions. This sort of disharmony represents a major road block to you receiving life's precious gifts and then giving those gifts to others. Make it easy for your life to go well by being consistent about how you give to yourself and others.

We all regularly benefit from the generosity of others and often don't even know when someone has extended a kindness to us. Some people call these folks angels on earth; others call them compassionate, thoughtful people. When someone removes stray nails from the street and throws them in a trash can where they cannot puncture your car tires, your bicycle tires, or your foot, their gift to you is their ability to anticipate and prevent an unfortunate consequence of nails lying in the street.

I use this example of a simple act to demonstrate how very ordinary, perhaps unseen acts can help total strangers every day of our lives. It is a joy to the person who picked up the nails to be of service in this way; they are not looking for thanks or a big parade. They know they have helped someone else have a better day simply because they took the time to remove something that could at the least interfere with most people's schedules.

Giving Your Money—Does It Always Make Sense?

There is more to the heart of giving than simply writing a check. Give of yourself in a way that honors you and those you wish to help. If giving your time means you will neglect your duties to yourself, your family, or others who rely on you in appropriate ways, then reconsider donating your time. If you have financial debts, you may need to learn to give to yourself first monetarily and fill that money hole before you give financial donations to others. Be mindful to give in ways that help you and help others; do not give at the expense of yourself. That is not what giving is about. Giving is sharing the extra in your life with others, not robbing from yourself just so you can say you gave. This discretion is part of personal integrity and congruence. Helen, whose story follows, learned this lesson well as she faced a time of financial difficulty.

Note: Helen's story is a composite based on multiple experiences. The rest of the following stories are true, but the names of the people have been changed to protect their privacy.

Helen's Story

Helen always made it a habit to give to her church no matter what. She gave a minimum of 20 percent of her income, and if she did not have 20 percent one week she made up for it the next week. She wanted to give to others and to things she believed in, but she wasn't aware that she also needed to give to herself.

Sometimes Helen's bills hit all at once. She also had a hard time handling unexpected major expenses, such as a new roof on her home. She dreaded these times when it seemed that everything needed to be paid, but she just didn't have the money to do it.

Helen was in tears the day she needed a new pair of custom orthopedic shoes, her home needed a new roof, and her daughter's tuition bill needed to be paid. She had no idea how she would come up with the needed money so quickly. She also knew that if she delayed paying for the most expensive item, the roof repair, her home would suffer massive water damage.

Helen valued her daughter's education above everything else, and she didn't want to have to pull her daughter from school while she came up with the money for tuition. Then there were her shoes. As a nurse at a big hospital, she worked on her feet all day (and sometimes all night), often working overtime so she could make more money. Having neglected her feet before, Helen knew that if she did not replace her shoes, she would have more foot and back trouble, miss work, and lose income.

Helen felt completely overwhelmed. Then she realized that since she had no way to increase her income, she had to cut expenses; the family income—her nursing paycheck and her daughter's paper route earnings—only went so far. She began to look closely where their money went. Though her daughter saved some of her paper route earnings, she spent most of it on "fun" things like candy and comic books. Helen's paycheck paid the taxes and their mortgage; purchased groceries, utilities, haircuts, beauty salon treatments, manicures and pedicures, and the latest clothes. In addition to the 20 percent she tithed to her church, she donated money to every charitable cause that came along. She was really proud of her giving spirit, and she loved the feeling this display of wealth and generosity gave her.

As Helen tracked their expenses, she realized that important family needs—such as the roof repair, her new shoes, and her daughter's tuition—were last on the "to be paid" list. Helen remembered hearing the saying "pay yourself first," but she hadn't really grasped what it might mean for her. Now it was clearer, much clearer, as she reviewed their overall finances.

But right now, she still had to deal with the roof, her daughter's tuition, and her shoes. First, she went to the hospital credit union and asked for a home equity loan to cover the cost of the roof repair. She didn't really want to borrow money, but she knew if the roof weren't repaired, she would end up spending even more. Then she called her daughter's school to work out a tuition payment plan. Once the roof and the tuition were handled, she had enough left in her checking account to pay for her shoes.

Next Helen tackled her ongoing finances. She reorganized how she paid her bills, investigated how to pay off her mortgage earlier, and put her charitable giving on a budget. (She realized that she was not a bad person for taking care of herself and her family first; she could then share with others at a level that made sense for her family.) Helen also opened a savings account for emergencies and unexpected expenses. She and her daughter made a game of who could save the most money (on a percentage basis, since her daughter made much less than she did). They looked at the money each of them spent, how necessary it really was to spend it, and then how much joy it gave them to spend it. Helen's stress around paying bills melted away because their whole financial situation was no longer a mystery to her, and she finally stopped worrying that they would not make it if she suddenly could no longer work at full capacity.

Helen's borderline high blood pressure (142/93 mm Hg) came down to normal and stayed there as she took firm control of her finances. It had another benefit as well: her elevated cholesterol and triglyceride levels dropped to normal. What does budgeting have to do with nutrition, you ask? Lots. For many people, these two are closely tied together. Helen noticed that she consistently spent over $400 a month on fast food. Her ongoing excuses were "I'm too busy to cook" or "I deserve a treat after a hard day's work" or "I'm going to do something for myself today even if it kills me, girl!" Also, her feet really did hurt at times, and it was just too painful to be standing up cooking, cleaning, and dealing with kitchen chores.

As a nurse, Helen knew she couldn't continue to ignore all the extra fat in her diet. She had seen plenty of people, especially Black women, in the hospital near death's door due to heart troubles. She did not want to be like one of her patients—lying in the hospital after a stroke or a heart attack for weeks, trying to recover their health and go on with their lives—so she began to change her eating habits.

The family bill for eating out plummeted as Helen and her daughter prepared meals together. Helen emphasized steamed vegetables and fresh salads, which her daughter could prepare. She also grilled, baked, or poached seafood, poultry, or meats in batches to save time and lower the electricity bill. (They cooked for an hour twice a week to prepare food for the whole week.)

Helen was very pleased with the choices she now was making. She understood her former habits and knew she could make positive changes in her life. She also knew she was teaching her daughter valuable life lessons: healthy food preparation skills and good eating habits as well as better habits and values concerning money. Including her daughter in managing family finances and in cooking sessions had another benefit. One day her daughter showed Helen information on the Internet about the difference between *saving* your money and *investing* your money. This idea of investing was new for Helen, and it opened her eyes as to why for years she'd felt she couldn't get ahead of her bills. She began researching mutual funds and other financial vehicles, and then she began investing money from every paycheck. In an account designed for minors, her daughter did the same with the earnings from her paper route. Together they reviewed their investments regularly, thinking of them as financial checkups and fiscal fitness exams.

Both Helen and her daughter also came to regard their changes in nutrition as investments in themselves. Their lives were never the same once they realized these relationships about giving to yourself first. It really does allow you to give more to others once you have taken care of what you need for you. There are no substitutes for this. They gave themselves really nutritious food, great beliefs and actions about health and wealth, and practical ways to invest that supported them in what they needed. Their willingness to keep what was working well in their lives and get rid of what was not serving a useful purpose allowed them to participate in helping others in ways that were mutually beneficial.

Giving to Yourself in Ways That Serve You

There is another aspect to giving that I have observed many times in my patients. For some people, health issues are directly related to money issues. These people have a tough time giving to themselves in ways that really matter. They will spend money on eating out, fancy clothes, cars, and other assets of dubious value before they will spend money on things that allow them to take better care of themselves. Often these are the very folks who can afford to do better on their own behalf. Issues around health and money are tied together so that improvement in one area usually leads to needed changes in the other area.

Laura's Story

I remember well a patient I encountered when I was just about finished with my clinical training in naturopathic medical school. Laura seemed quite excited and upbeat as we began the office visit that day, saying that she had received a raise in her pay at work, she was feeling better overall, her primary health complaints were steadily improving, and she had bought a new car. Laura was really starting to feel good and enjoy her life again. But toward the end of the appointment, she complained about having to pay for her health care and started going off about the costs of treatment. She became verbally abusive about having to pay for her care. This behavior caught me off guard, as it seemed so out of place with everything else that was going on in the context of her health care and her life in general.

Now here Laura was, making use of a teaching clinic where visits cost about $15. She had just purchased a new car, gotten a raise, and, most importantly, was getting and enjoying a return of her health. I was amazed to hear her complain. Something about what she had said just did not sit right with me. I realized that she was not upset with me personally and that she probably felt safe enough with me to let loose some of her distress about this aspect of life. I felt she was asking for help in a round-about way, so I took the plunge and responded.

I began by saying that I could not be both her doctor and her financial planner. It is a moral hazard to recommend to patients care based on their ability to pay versus presenting them with the optimal treatment plan, which of course they may amend as they wish based on their financial situation. I simply cannot make that call. If I recommend less care than is needed and, God forbid, my patient suffers because of it, we both lose. It is a boundary I cannot cross. It is the patient's body and health, so the patient must be in charge of how to respond financially to health care needs.

I reminded Laura that health care costs do not get much cheaper than they are at a teaching clinic, and that by her own admission she was getting what she came for in terms of health results. If she was not satisfied or thought she could do better elsewhere, I was willing to transfer her records as appropriate once she signed a release of records request. I also pointed out that with this newfound health, her work performance had improved, thus allowing her to get a raise and buy a new car. Not bad for the cost of her visits to the teaching clinic, huh? I then said that she should really consider if the key issue was the money spent on her health because, frankly, its total cost to date could only represent a fraction of her monthly car payments. She looked at me and blinked a couple times. The room was silent for a while. Laura said, "Let me think about what you just said." I said "OK," and we finished our office visit. After she left, I thought about what I had said too, wondering if I had been inappropriate, if I should have ignored her, or if I had said what she really needed to hear.

When Laura came for her next appointment, I had my answer. We sat down together in the treatment room and she looked at me with a sheepish smile on her face. She thanked me for my comments, said they really hit home and that since our conversation, she had found a fee-only financial planner who was helping her get her money and investment plans in order. She was also starting to get counseling about her issues with money. She realized that she had delayed getting any health care until she could no longer ignore her symptoms. Had she been willing earlier to spend some money on behalf of her health, she would not have been in such bad shape when she initially came in and probably would have needed to spend less to regain her health. Laura realized that these decisions and behaviors were part of a pattern of her neglecting her own needs and then blaming others for her troubles. Laura had her break-through! I was pleased for her and relieved that my willingness to say what I felt was the truth had turned into something wonderful for my patient. My comments sparked her to make better decisions concerning her health and her money. In a later office visit toward the end of her care, Laura told me that was the first time anyone had stood up to her about her stuff with money. I was glad I had taken a chance to counsel her about the relationship between her upset with her finances and the state of her health.

Barbara's Story

Barbara, a woman in her early fifties, made an appointment to see me because she had some health problems as well as some money problems. She was on welfare and was a single parent trying to raise her teenage son. Her health problems revolved around difficulties with menopause; drenching sweats at night; skin, hair, and nail troubles; and problems with her concentration.

When she came for her first appointment, she arrived about one hour late. After we finished, I told her what I thought would be involved in helping her restore her health. When she was presented with the charges for her office visit and physical examination, she balked. She did not want to pay and felt her visit should be free and that future visits should be free too. After all, she told me, her money was tight. I asked her if her housing for herself and her son was free, she said no; I asked if their food and the fuel for her car were free. Again, she replied no. I then said "Well, my time and skills are not free either." She was late to the ap-pointment, did not call to say she was delayed, and seemed eager to make her financial difficulties my problem.

During the initial office visit and exam, it was clear that she was in the habit of making her problems other people's problems. She wouldn't even take steps to see to it that she and her son regularly had food but instead chose to rely on neighbors and acquaintances to bring food by from their gardens. Anytime someone is willing to settle for an unpredictable food source rather than see to it this gets handled in a reliable fashion, you know something significant is happening.

Taking into account everything that I had learned about Barbara, coupled with prior experiences, I knew that it was not going to work well for me or anyone else to be her doctor until she stepped up to this money issue. Her neglect of her physical health was reflected in her neglect of her financial health and other aspects of responsibility in her life. I'd already worked with several patients who were on welfare, work disability, or other kinds of limited income who somehow found a way to pay cash out of pocket and never made their money problems an issue for me or my staff. They were clear about their financial responsibilities. In fact, one man who was out on disability got angry when I offered to treat him for free, feeling that he would be taking a handout and that was against his beliefs; he valued my skills and services and was paying, end of story. So with these other experiences in my mind, I considered my options for possible responses.

Here is what I said to Barbara: "You do have to pay for this first visit. We did not agree in advance of this appointment to some other financial arrangement, but you knew that this was not a free clinic. What you have shared of your health history indicates a chronic pattern of self-neglect, and it is deeply affecting your quality of life and that of your son's. You need to make some changes for things to get better, as you are depleted in more than just nutrients at this time. I do not think I am a good fit for you as a doctor. I only take patients I sincerely believe I can help and who really want help. It appears to me that there is an imbalance here. I am concerned that your issues with money are a way you show a lack of respect for yourself and others. If you would like some suggestions for referrals, I would be happy to provide them. Think about what you want to do and let me know." She was upset at first and tried to defend her behavior. I remained steadfast. She paid and left, and that was the last I heard of her.

I truly hope Barbara got her life together again. No one deserves to needlessly struggle like that. As a doctor, it is a judgment call to know when to offer a financial break to a patient if it is at all possible. We have bills to pay, employee payroll to meet, and other financial obligations that either severely limit or make it impossible to treat people for free. In my opinion, attitude is everything in these cases. My observation is that when people come to the healing environment with a heart full of riches, even when their financial situation does not reflect their inner wealth, they regain their health faster and are better able to share that experience with others. They are coming from a place of fullness, not lack. Folks who come from a place of "the glass is half empty" often have more work to do to regain their health. It is interesting to watch these dynamics play out in people's lives. Most of us hit a rough patch in life now and again. How we handle it makes all the difference in the quality of life we lead. We determine for ourselves our approach to handling difficulties and adversities. We choose our responses to challenges.

Not to belabor the point, but if you recognize yourself in any of these people for whom issues about money and health were tied together, please address this promptly. Pull yourself out of the trap of this kind of unworkable thinking. One of the best gifts you can ever give yourself is to get free of mental and spiritual shackles. Your beliefs determine your actions and your actions determine your results. Beware of taking on any identities of illness, lack, helplessness, or unworthiness. These kinds of identities keep you stuck in insidious old ways of behaving and thinking. They are sneaky traps that you do not deserve to be stuck in.

Julie's Story

Another patient, Julie, stands out in my mind because she continued to amaze me throughout our work together in restoring her formerly robust health. Julie walked away from a high-powered, very stressful, and extremely well-paying job that she came to realize was killing her. Her realization came on her vacation to several undeveloped countries where she could see the impact of the decisions she made in her work every day. The poverty she saw on her trip was at a level she had not known was still possible in the modern world. Julie realized how insulated she was from these people and the results of the decisions she made as a routine part of her work. When she returned from vacation, the incongruence between what she had just visited and the stamp her work left on the world caused her to abruptly quit her job. She had a nervous breakdown and left the big city, heading for a remote area in an attempt to come to terms with herself and her former job.

When Julie came to my clinic, she was on welfare and insisted that she could pay for treatment; she valued what I had to offer and said she would find a way to come up with the money. She had been in and out of mental institutions over the last several years and was trying to avoid a return trip to yet another one. She very much wanted to find paying work she could do, but the local economy was not strong, and jobs that paid decent wages were hard to find.

Her physical, mental, emotional, and spiritual symptoms were intense and deep seated. As I worked with Julie, sometimes it was not always clear what the cause or source of her symptoms was, so as we went along, her feedback was invaluable in providing me the clues I needed to help her get the job done. As her doctor, I had my work cut out for me in determining what realm her symptoms really came from. Part of the joy of working with natural therapies is that they are so very flexible and allow me as a naturopathic physician to tailor treatment plans to individuals and not just try to treat disease entities. At one point, Julie had an episode of severe upper abdominal pain that represented a worsening disturbance in her liver and gallbladder function and digestion of fatty foods. I had to determine if this pain was an acute gallbladder attack (gallstones) or a disruption of her gallbladder meridian (from the point of view of traditional Chinese medicine). I sent her off for some diagnostic imaging; the abdominal ultrasound revealed she was fine on the physical plane. With the worry of a possible gallbladder rupture removed, I then treated her for the disturbed meridian, and all symptoms associated with it resolved. In situations like these, it is great to be able to use the best of both the modern and ancient worlds in the service of people's health.

During one of her first visits, Julie said she felt as if her heart was breaking. She felt deep remorse and guilt that anyone should have to live in the squalor she had seen on her trip to these developing countries. Julie felt that the world was not a fair place, and she felt helpless to make a positive difference. She had "night terrors," as she called them, where her dreams became nightmares revolving around her childhood and the lack of genuine love and warmth from her parents. She was the oldest child and often chose to intervene when her parents, both alcoholics, started severely beating her brothers. Julie would then be the one they beat.

As she went through the course of treatment, she had a series of profound breakthroughs that totally turned around her physical health and her mental attitude concerning her role in life, her purpose in this world. She got a job as a part-time bookkeeper and accountant, decided to quit smoking, and realized that she first had to accept her past and let it go, all of it. In her opinion, the best thing she could do with her past was learn from it and move on. Loving herself was now central to developing into the woman she wanted to be in the world. She needed to accept all parts of herself, including embracing her flaws as well as the aspects of her self that she was pleased with. Julie was consciously becoming a person who added value to the world in all realms and was actively holding it out as a possibility for others who might be feeling trapped in their lives. She began volunteering in the community with grassroots organizations, sharing with others some of the lessons she had learned about making life go well for herself and others. She became much more able to accept the love and support of her husband, who kept encouraging her over the years to seek out treatment that would be effective for her.

At our last office visit at the end of her treatment program, she told me she was at peace from the inside out for the first time in a long time. I was touched by her courage to face her life honestly and go forward making changes as she could. She did not let the fact that it was easier to make excuses for her situation be the way she let her life play out. Just as it was for Julie, reaching for your own personal power is always a marvelous thing to do.

Giving Your Time and Skills as a Volunteer

Many people serve as volunteers. These folks do a great service to us all as they make available their time, talents, love, and caring to help the lives of others go well. These contributions really make a difference for organizations and the people they serve. This generosity of spirit goes forth in the world, spreading good cheer and easing the loads others carry. Volunteers should always be thanked and appreciated for their efforts. These people are a delightful part of the circle of life.

Have you considered being a volunteer? Can you volunteer your time, energy, skills, or money to a cause or person in need? What do you want for yourself from the experience of giving to others in this way? What do you want others to experience as a result of your gift?

Vivian's Story

Life had given Vivian many major setbacks, and she rebounded every time. Some recoveries from difficult life events took longer than others, yet when it was all said and done, she never gave up hope of having her life the way she wanted it. Vivian, being a very thoughtful person, loved to help others and genuinely offered her time, skills, energy, and love without expectation of a lot in return; a heartfelt "thank you" or some other simple acknowledgment was sufficient.

Vivian volunteered for her own reasons. It was not to impress anyone or to be viewed as a "do-gooder." Volunteering was her way of giving back God's blessings in life. Vivian was well aware that she had experienced her share of down times and hardships. Now that she was retired, she had her time to herself to use as she pleased. Since her retirement income took care of her financial needs, she knew she had the resources to be helpful and supportive of others. For Vivian, it was personally fulfilling to be of service. She felt strong spiritual gratification in helping those in need. She chose to work with teenagers, showing them how to sail boats and experience a different slice of life than they had access to in their families and neighborhoods. The other place she focused her volunteering efforts was at her church, doing such good works as taking Holy Communion to the sick and those unable to travel to church. She also did some bookkeeping and other administrative tasks to take some of the load off the clerical staff at the rectory.

Vivian makes it a point to help wherever she feels she is needed most, or as she puts it, she goes "where the Lord tells me I can best help."

She consciously asks the Holy Spirit for guidance and gets still within herself, waiting for the response. Now she only goes where Spirit leads her. Vivian said that she found her volunteering efforts did not turn out well or feel good to her if she forced the situation or picked a volunteer position for what she felt were the wrong reasons. When Vivian felt that inner tug to offer help, the situation flowed well; when the inner voice was absent, the situation did not go well.

I find this an interesting observation. Many times my patients have told me that when they feel they are "in the zone" or "in the flow" of honoring what they feel is part of their life's purpose, all sorts of situations work out and miracles occur on a regular basis. These same people have commented that when they force something, really push to make it happen, whatever they were working so hard to create unravels, just falls apart like it wasn't supposed to be that way in the first place.

Patients and friends of mine who express fulfillment with their lives share at least one common trait: they know when to insist on something and when to let go. This important distinction between doing something because it is what needs to be done versus doing it because we will it to be so, really highlights the difference between doing things for reasons of ego and doing things for reasons that transcend self, surrendering to the will of Spirit. You just cannot buy this kind of peace of mind and peace of spirit. It nourishes and sustains an unshakable inner smile. No one and nothing can keep people with this attitude from eventually seeing the good in a situation and finding their own way to inner peace and harmony. From this spiritual place of plenty, the volunteer can effectively share with others, because she knows she has enough. As I have said before, love is an inside job, as Vivian knew well.

Over time, as Vivian's experiences as a volunteer grew, she found that she liked the freedom to contribute where she felt most needed and that if things did not work out, she could end it and go elsewhere. At first in her early volunteer experiences, Vivian would go in to a situation expecting one thing and sometimes find out that things were not as they appeared in the beginning. As a rookie volunteer, she felt obligated to stick it out, but she later realized that she did not have to do this. She learned it was important not to allow herself to be stretched beyond her limits; she had to say "no" when her own boundaries or ability to give were being pushed too far. For Vivian, part of her success formula as a volunteer was to do simple things that were appreciated. She also learned how much time she could give without jeopardizing her own self-care. Performing volunteer activities once or twice a week fit her schedule—physically, mentally, emotionally, and spiritually— quite well.

Vivian learned that one of the keys to having a satisfying experience as a volunteer was to find a good match between what someone else needed and what she felt she could do. The best volunteer experiences matched Vivian's needs and ability to assist. For Vivian, helping out and knowing she made someone else's life easier provided her with deep satisfaction. And it was fun! Her advice to others considering being volunteers is to find something you enjoy and give it a try. If it does not work, it's no problem. Since your work as a volunteer is not set in stone, just move on until you find something where your contribution feels good to you and is good for others too. That is the match you are looking for as a volunteer. This generates lots of goodwill and can inspire others to share their resources as volunteers too. Vivian was very grateful to God for the opportunity to share her gifts with others. Being a volunteer can touch the lives of others, and it will touch your life in return. Try it—you'll see!

The Heart of Courage

Courage takes many forms in our lives. It takes courage to do what you know is right even when it is not convenient. Courage is required when you step out in new directions in your life, perhaps going into territory that is unfamiliar to you, your family, and your friends. Many acts of courage occur every day without fanfare or acknowledgment. I offer some examples for your consideration.

When single parents care for their children in a responsible manner, despite one missing parent (for whatever reason), and see to it that their obligations to the children are fulfilled, that takes courage. Many parents feel that there are not enough hours in the day to get everything done. But for single parents, there is even more to do in less time. It takes courage to do the right thing, even when it seems impossible.

Courage is displayed whenever you choose to be yourself in the face of peer pressure. Courage is evident when you admit your mistakes and shortcomings to others and make amends as needed to those who have been harmed. It takes courage to forgive others for harm they have caused you, and courage to insist that those who have caused you harm face the consequences of their behaviors. It takes courage to love again after the loss of a major love relationship, and courage must be summoned so you can trust again after a significant betrayal by someone you considered to be part of your inner circle of friends and confidantes. If you stop and think about it, there are many examples of courage in each of our lives.

What are some acts of courage you remember that bring a smile to your lips and a song to your heart? What makes them such great examples of courage for you?

Now let's look at courage from a different perspective. Do you shrink from life's challenges, or face them squarely? Do you make excuses for yourself or others? Do you accept the past for what it is— the past—or do you allow yourself to dwell on it longer than necessary? Identify what keeps you from the prudent use of your own courage, your own personal power, and remove it as soon as you can. Again, it has been my experience that most of us know what we need to do in our lives but neglect to do it.

Earlier in this book, I spoke of the need for emotional closure around unfinished business and how unfinished business can be an obstacle to the development of outstanding heart health. Clean out your closet of regrets and disappointments about things long since over and done with. Let in the fresh air and sunshine so you can grow and thrive. In its own way, getting rid of clutter (of any kind) takes courage. And one act of courage often leads to other acts of courage— our own and others. Courage is an act of the heart, and we seek to be heart healthy in every way. Jeffrey, who was a patient of mine, is a wonderful example of this.

Jeffrey's Story

Jeffrey is one of the most remarkable people it has ever been my privilege to work with. Although Jeffrey is a man, I include his story here because it exemplifies so many of the elements of healing with respect to heart disease. Jeffrey had congestive heart failure; coccidiomycosis; pronounced spinal scoliosis; a chronically very low body temperature; and an emotional past filled with two abusive, alcoholic parents, an alcoholic, bipolar ex-wife, and three children he loved dearly but didn't always quite know how to handle (a feeling shared by many parents).

Jeffrey's health had been in decline for decades. At the local teaching hospital for a conventional medical school, he had been placed on the heart transplant list, as his heart pumped too little blood to meet the needs of his body. If a donor organ became available, his cardiologist wanted him to get a transplant. In fact, when I met him, he was number one on the heart transplant list.

During our initial meeting, he emphatically stated that he did not want a heart transplant, since this procedure would mean he would have to remain on pharmaceutical drugs that suppressed his immune system for most, if not all, of his lifetime. Jeffrey was interested in pursuing any other means of treatment, if it meant he could keep his original heart. He asked what the possibilities for treatments from the realm of natural health care were, as he felt those remedies and treatments would be safer and less invasive than transplantation. He also wondered if it would be possible for me to coordinate care with his conventional medical doctors, especially his cardiologist, as he was concerned about possible adverse side effects or interactions between the natural treatments and the pharmaceutical drugs. He had already experienced complications from some of his prescription pharmaceutical drugs, where the side effects had masked the worsening of some symptoms of congestive heart failure. I told him that I was quite willing to coordinate care and that we would have to see how the cardiologist responded, as he might or might not welcome the addition of a different medical approach. I assured Jeffrey I would do all I could to cooperate but reminded him that cooperation is a two-way street.

As I got to know Jeffrey better, he confided in me extensively about his past, the personal history that plagued him so at times. The details he shared about his emotional and spiritual worlds made it clear that even if all of his heart symptoms were resolved, there would still be echoes from his past that put him at risk of losing whatever health gains he had made in the course of our work together. He needed to heal emotionally, no matter what happened physically.

Jeffrey's emotional past provided rich clues to what was troubling him spiritually and mentally. He spent his childhood with abusive, alcoholic, unreliable parents. Those family dynamics set the stage for many of his later struggles. As he grew to adulthood, there were times when he could no longer stand being around his alcoholic parents, and he despaired that things would never change. One particular episode, which happened when he was 18, haunted him still, some thirty-odd years later. One Christmas Eve, a time when the world was supposed to be full of good cheer and love for one another, Jeffrey tried unsuccessfully to kill his

Tips for Eating Healthily in the Real World

Money Stress

Focus on low-cost, high-nutrition foods such as fresh vegetables, whole grains, beans, peas, brown rice (the fiber on the rice hulls is what makes this rice brown and good for your blood sugar, cholesterol level, and colon too), tofu, sprouts, and fruits in season. Good nutrition does not have to cost a fortune. Buy generic brands instead of brands that have a large marketing budget. In numerous cases, the generic items are the same as the name brands. Factories often have deals where they relabel their products as the house brand so as to appear to increase the competition. The money all goes to the same place—the factory—and leaves from the same place—your wallet. Be creative in how you save money by reducing the costs of eating while increasing the quality of what you eat. Make choices that support your health and wealth at the same time. Consider outdoor exercise over joining a club if you can't afford fees and dues. Used exercise equipment costs much less than brand new and may make it more convenient for you to exercise at home. Grow your own food in a garden. Walk instead of driving to destinations in your neighborhood.

parents and then commit suicide. That was a day, he told me, he could never forget, nor would he forgive himself for trying to kill his parents and himself. He was in tears while he recounted this sad moment in his life, a time when he just could not think of what else to do to deal with the situation he found himself in. He wanted to end once and for all his parents' physical and verbal abuse of him and his brothers and sisters, as well as their incessant drinking and carousing.

Shortly after the attempted murder and suicide, Jeffrey moved out of his parents' home and went out on his own. He joined the Army for a few years and met a woman with whom he fell deeply in love; they married and had three children together. After much pleading and cajoling, Jeffrey finally got his wife to the doctor, where they learned she suffered from bipolar disorder (formerly called manic-depression) along with alcoholism. With three young children to raise, Jeffrey at first thought he should stick it out with his wife for the sake of the children. He was not eager to be divorced and raising three children by himself. However, it became clear that he and the children were better off without her. He filed for divorce, feeling very much that everything and everyone he touched somehow suffered.

Ever since that traumatic Christmas Eve, Jeffrey had been unconsciously punishing himself for what he had tried to do to his parents and to himself by creating a crisis of some sort at the holidays. As one of his teenage children told me during an office visit, it was their family tradition to react to whatever emotional vortex Dad stirred up or got involved in during the holiday season. They usually wound up at the emergency room, the police station, or a crisis intervention center in their community as their dad went through his holiday ritual. Jeffrey had not consciously realized that this pattern of behavior during the holidays might be tied to his earlier attempt to murder his parents and himself. Having been raised Catholic, he was distinctly aware of the prohibition against taking a human life. He felt awful about what he had tried to do that Christmas Eve so many years ago. He felt that he did not deserve to enjoy the time of Christmas at all.

Jeffrey's heart health had worsened during his young-adult and middle-age years, steadily eroding until it was hard for him to take a full breath or walk much more than 50 steps before he became winded and very tired. He was now 52; he was first diagnosed with congestive heart failure when he was 45. It had been observed on x-rays taken in his early twenties that his heart was abnormally large (left ventricular hypertrophy) and that the heart walls were on the thin side, indicating that his enlarged heart was not due to an athletic history but to a disease process. Over the years, various doctors warned him that his condition would probably worsen, because eventually his body would no longer compensate for the fact that his heart was literally too big. Ironically, Jeffrey had confided that he did not know how to keep anything back for himself, that all he knew how to do was give. He realized he was out of balance and that perhaps his physical state of health mirrored his mental and emotional state of health. He wondered if in his case his overly large heart was a physical metaphor for a behavioral pattern that was slowly and steadily killing him.

With Jeffrey's complex and multifaceted health history, it was critical to treat the whole person. We began with very gradual changes in his level of physical activity and a strong program of specific botanical (herbal) medicines and nutritional supplements designed to replace potassium, stimulate normal kidney function, promote diuresis (decreasing edema through increased kidney function and urination), lower his high blood pressure, and nourish his heart muscle tissue. These were coupled with emotional counseling. Jeffrey made tangible progress that was verified by his subjective reporting of how he felt and what his daily activity levels were. Objective lab tests measured things like how much blood his heart was pumping and the efficiency with which it pumped the blood. Toward the end of the initial treatment period, Jeffrey suffered a major setback in the form of two strokes in the course of a week. Now he had slurred speech, facial droop, and foot drop that persisted for months. Slowly he began to show signs of steady progress during his recovery and rehabilitation. To his credit, Jeffrey did not let the strokes discourage him. He simply refused to quit or give up. He really wanted as much health back as he could muster. After about seven months, he was back to where he had been before the strokes and from that place, he got really excited about what health recovery might be possible for him. He became more willing to make indicated changes to his nutrition. Until that time, he felt that nutrition was not a big factor in his healing process, feeling much more that quality time with his doctor was what mattered; he felt he had a very caring connection with me. Jeffrey thought of love as a nutrient; in fact, he called love the most important ingredient in life.

Our work together continued on all fronts—physical, emotional, and spiritual. Jeffrey's extremely high blood pressure improved over the course of treatment, as the herbal medicines and nutritional supplements helped nourish his physical cardiovascular system and counseling about his demons from the past helped heal his emotional heart. After I realized what the Christmas holiday meant to him, we worked together to give him very specific homework he had to do during the course of the season so that he would really understand that he did not have to keep on torturing himself for past mistakes. It was time for him to enjoy life, and he had to start by forgiving his parents for who they were and forgiving himself for what he had tried to do to them and to himself.

That first Christmas season we worked together was a breakthrough for him. For the first time since he was 18, he really had fun in the month of December, and his children felt they had a new dad. Jeffrey told me that there were times when he did not know what to do with himself during the holidays, since there was no crisis to occupy his time and divert his attention. He even spent a day with his ex-wife, and they did not argue like they usually did when they were together. During the time between Thanksgiving and New Year's Day, I had him plan out how he would handle the emotional triggers he knew about and what he would do if he discovered anything new that would tug him toward feeling bad and trying to create chaos as he had in the past. I had him do things like play Santa Claus at a children's home, volunteer at a Salvation Army depot, make a list of all the people in his life he was grateful for, write letters to people he cared about, and find things at home to give away to others. I also encouraged him to resume his work with A Course in Miracles, as he felt it had helped him tremendously.

By the time we were done working together intensively on his heart health, Jeffrey was no longer on the heart transplant list. His high blood pressure was under control, he was no longer retaining water, his initial shortness of breath was gone, and he could go through a normal day without becoming overly tired. He found parenting was easier when he had more energy. His stamina had improved dramatically, as he easily walked up, down, and around a hill near his neighborhood. All of these changes took place in a man who could barely make it from the front door of the clinic to the nearest treatment room when I first met him. I was so pleased to help him get his life back in order, and I learned a ton from him. He taught me that all things are possible as long as we think they are possible. Whenever I think of Jeffrey, I am reminded that there is a reason why we call a doctor's work a "practice." I easily learned as much as, if not more than, I taught, while working with Jeffrey.

The Heart of Grace

Moments of grace in our lives can be times when we feel most in touch with our Creator. These are the times when you feel tingles down your spine because you are so emotionally moved by something you've experienced, seen, or heard. Often people have few or no words for their experiences of grace, as they can be intensely personal; recalling the scenes can bring tears to their eyes.

People who are considered "gracious" are often skilled at putting others at ease or being diplomatic during tough situations. These folks bring out the best in the people in their lives and exemplify "a touch of class." Their behaviors and movements flow well with what is needed in the moment as they expertly say and do the things that keep harmony present. To be both gracious and graceful is to be doubly blessed.

How often in your life do you experience moments of grace? Is it daily, weekly, or a couple of times a year? Have you had experiences when your heart and soul were stirred, when something touched your innermost being deeply and powerfully and all your worries and concerns faded, with not even so much as a wisp of fretting left over? Some of us have these experiences when we are out in nature and enjoy the beauty of a bird's song; when we stroll through our neighborhood and hear delight in a child's voice; or during times of prayer and meditation, when the mind, body, and spirit are all quiet at the same time.

Would you feel your life were as rich if you never experienced any moments of grace? Grace touches our hearts and speaks to us in ways that are beyond the ordinary appeal of common things. Grace—though generally uncommon—is precious.

The Heart of Loving

Ah, love. What a special, magnificent feeling love is! When your heart is swept up in an emotional bond in which you feel fulfilled, when you really look forward to being with someone else, and when that person occupies a special place in your mind and spirit, you are indeed in love. There are no substitutes for loving someone and being loved by another person. Many women say that they feel differently about their world and about themselves when they have a satisfying love relationship. Much more seems possible when we are in love; this is especially true when we love ourselves. In fact, we have much more love to give when our own "love tank" is filled, nourished from within. Too many people look to others for love, thinking that someone or something outside of them will give them the love they seek. These people are not looking in the right place. Love is, first and foremost, an inside job.

What does love mean to you? How do you know when you feel love? How do you know when someone else loves you? If you feel that love is missing in your life, examine your approach to love, how you give it and receive it. If you are too picky, you may miss out on other people's attempts to love you in ways that are different from how you may want to be loved. You may not even notice the way love flows to you; perhaps your focus is on what's missing rather than what is present.

These shifts in perception are powerful and subtle at the same time. They are powerful in that a change in perspective can quickly and dramatically improve your perception of your quality of life, seemingly overnight in some cases. These shifts in perception are subtle; they do not usually require huge alterations, just incremental course corrections as you go along in your primary relationships.

Consider whether there is room in your life to allow more opportunities for love. Do your current behaviors and daily activities have enough slack in them for unscheduled moments of love? Are you in frequent enough contact with the people you love that they know you love them? Are they in contact with you on a frequent enough basis that you know they love you? When you are in contact with people you love, is the encounter a quality experience for both of you? When it comes to love, many of us choose quality over quantity, as our needs for satisfaction and fulfillment are better met with a few quality loving relationships than with multiple superficial relationships where the love between the parties may constantly be in question.

Take time to assess the flow of love in your life. If you're giving out more love than you feel you receive, step back and check out why that may be the case. Ask yourself if maybe you are giving too much, more than makes sense.

Or maybe you are making it difficult for others to give you love? If you make it hard for others to give you love, but you are unaware that you are doing this, you may feel either unloved or empty inside, as my patient Sheila did.

Sheila's Story

I remember working with Sheila on her issues about love and how she felt it was impacting her overall health. As she spoke, tears welled up in her eyes when she described how she felt she was all alone and that no one really cared.

When I asked her to describe in more detail how she came to these conclusions, it became clear that the way she currently ran her life made it tough for others to have much chance to really connect with her and demonstrate their love in ways she could understand and appreciate. Sheila mapped out her "rules of love," and as she did the exercise, she recognized that it was just about impossible for anyone to get through both her emotional shell and the hectic pace at which she conducted her life.

This realization fortified her decision to make a big change in her life. She resolved to create the life of her dreams and transform anything that stood in her way of getting what she wanted. She realized that there were likely to be both welcome and unwelcome surprises, and she decided in advance she would see it through. Feeling unloved and feeling her heart was frozen simply was not worth the pain. She needed to move out of her comfort zone and risk future joys, disappointments, and other emotional unknowns.

Sheila made changes in her home life first, then in her workplace; finally, she carved out time for doing nothing at all and for being spontaneous, seeking new adventures when the mood struck her. She often expressed surprise at how differently other people were treating her now and commented on the large and small events that happened in her life just about every day that let her know she was loved by others. Since love is an inside job, Sheila came to realize that she had to love herself first and get familiar with what that felt like before she could fully recognize the love other people gave her.

Her overall health improved significantly, and Sheila found it easier as time went by to make the connection between her emotional health and her physical health. What she had at first thought were unrelated parts of her life, she now came to realize were intimately woven together. Changes in her physical health had impact in the spiritual realm, and changes in attitude shifted her behavior and choices so that it was possible for more love to come into her life.

Sheila also noted that the kind of people she spent her free time with shifted too. Her friends became more loving people, and now, she does not think of her family members in such rigid ways; they in turn have softened their responses to her.

When people like Sheila understand at their core how truly interconnected our lives are, it has a ripple effect in the larger world we all live in. As one person heals from the inside out, others are healed too as they benefit from that person's decisions and actions to make their life go well. They see the results that someone like Sheila has obtained and decide they want some of that too, for themselves; they want to identify their personal obstacles and sources of confusion, get this stuff untangled, and then move on with their lives.

It is beautiful to watch this dynamic operate in people's lives. Most people are capable of accomplishing far more than they realize in the context of how they live their lives. I am so proud of and pleased for anyone who really grabs life's brass ring. I commend anyone who is willing to do the work necessary to lead the life of their dreams. It is my privilege as a naturopathic physician to assist these seekers in their journeys.

Little Things Matter

A number of times, I have mentioned that what you do on a daily basis determines your overall health. The little things in life really do matter; they have effects over time. To illustrate this point, I ask you the following question. Over the course of a month, which would you rather have: a dollar a day for 30 days, or to start the month with one penny and have that initial penny doubled each day of the month for 30 days?

What did you choose? If you went for the dollar a day choice, at the end of the month you would have $30. If you selected the penny doubled every day for a month, then at the end of the month you would have $5,368,709.12.

Surprised? There's no magic here, just the effect of compounding at work. Check it out: the doubled-penny choice starts out small—day 1 is $0.01, day 2 is $0.02, day 3 is $0.04, day 4 is $0.08 etc.; at day 10, your initial penny is now worth $5.12, at day 12 it is worth $20.48, and at day 13 it is worth $40.96. That may not seem impressive yet, but hang on. It gets better. At day 20, it is worth $5,242.88. By the end of the month, at day 30 it is worth $5,368,709.12. That's right, choosing the penny option results in over $5 million at the end of the same month when with the other choice, you could have had just $30.

When presented with choices like these in our lives, many of us opt for the easy way out or the sure thing. You can quickly calculate in your mind that starting with a dollar a day you will have $30 at the end of the month. The value of a penny doubled every day of the month requires some thought and calculation.

Our health works the same way. The easy way out is usually not the way that produces the greatest value to our overall health in the physical, mental, emotional, or spiritual realms. Take the time to plan your activities and review your choices to be sure that they really serve you in getting what you want.

When applied to the area of health, quick fixes and shortcuts mask symptoms rather than identify and treat causes. For this reason, they are rarely adequate long-term solutions. Do not cheat yourself out of the great results you deserve by skimping on your exercise habits, eating choices, level of rest, or any of the other things that keep you jazzed about life and feeling positive about yourself and others.

Stay on Track for the Long Term

The checklists in the appendix are provided to help you stay on track with your heart healthy habits. I recommend you use all of them for at least one year to assist you in your journey. The checklists can be used as milestones along the way, affirming what you are doing well and illuminating any areas that need reinforcement or change.

These checklists can be used as a rolling plan over time to keep you on track. With clear targets in mind, it's much easier to plot a course and reach the destination. Any journey is easier if you know why you want to go and have a road map. These tools can serve as reminders of the activities that you need to do on a regular basis to create the right environment for heart health. Use them to your best advantage. This is part of your gift to yourself.

Until We Meet Again . . .

Throughout this book, I have tried to make few or no assumptions about what you as the reader may or may not know. I hope I have been able to clarify some things for you, present new information, and reinforce the correct information you already have.

It is my privilege to help you understand more about some of the factors that affect heart health and what can be done to turn health problems into opportunities for healing, growth, and new discoveries. And believe me, they can be.

I hope you use this book as a resource, a treasure chest of ideas and actions that you can take today and every day to get the level of health you so richly deserve. You are your own best friend when it comes to your health; you choose whether you really are your best friend or your worst enemy by the choices and actions you take. You are the one who has to live with the results day after day.

I hope that this book provides you with the knowledge, support, and inspiration you need for your heart healthy journey.

May your heart be filled with joy and gladness. Invest in your health for a lifetime. It will pay you repeatedly throughout your life. Live long and live well!

Visualization Exercise

(Do this exercise with your eyes closed. Make a tape of the instructions and the exercise so you can keep your eyes closed while listening.)

Close your eyes. In your mind, see yourself in vivid detail with your current level of heart health. Now step forward in time and picture yourself with your future level of heart health, that's right, the level you want to experience for yourself. Notice how the positive changes you make in your daily habits add to your heart health. Let the pictures and the feelings associated with these changes and continuation of great habits grow stronger. Allow your imagination to show you how much better you'll feel, how much more love and joy and gratitude you will experience in your daily life. Let images pour over you of how you'll look and feel one month from now based on all the good things you do for your overall health, especially your heart health. Really feel these feelings, let the images flow. Now look at three months from today, then six months, one year, a year and a half, two years, three years, five years, 10 years, 15 years, 20 years, 25 years, 50 years from now. Keep the images and feelings flowing. Let your spirit soar as you savor these pictures and emotions.

How does it feel to be in your body? What do you notice? What do you feel yourself thinking? What do you hear yourself saying as you talk to yourself? What were the consequences of the great decisions you made daily about your health? How much more have you enjoyed your life because you had true health? What life experiences did you get to have because you were alive *and* well? What moments are forever etched on your soul as "precious" because you treated yourself and others well? Did your level of health have an impact on the people around you? What was the "ripple effect" of your healthy habits? View yourself as the center of a still lake; let each positive change you made in your health flow out from you and ripple toward the loved ones in your life, people from your past and present whom you love and future people whom you will love. Let all these good feelings wash over you, soak in them, and bask in the knowledge that you did make a positive difference for yourself. Take credit for your good work, faith, and commitment to enjoying a higher level of health and wellness. You deserve it; well done! Congratulations on your present and future level of health. (End of tape)

If you have great health now or are in the process of creating it, you will best benefit from visualization when you do it on a daily basis. This conditions your psyche, behavior, and nervous system to align with your stated and intended goals. It is helpful to get all aspects of yourself moving in the same direction. This helps eliminate self-sabotage.

Health is like anything else in our lives; we get what we focus on. The more compelling and real your visualizations are, the more you are drawn to fulfilling your destiny of excellent heart health and all that goes with it. Since the mind cannot tell the difference between events that have already occurred and the things we vividly imagine, harness the power inherent in your thoughts to serve you in moving toward the health results you seek and in moving away from the diseases and symptoms you don't want in your life.

It's up to you.

Questions for Your Health Care Providers

While reading this book, some of you have been thinking, "Well, why not leave all of this up to the doctor? After all, she knows what's best." This kind of thinking has many implications. For starters, it implies that you and your loved ones actually go to the doctor regularly for checkups and that you know what's important to tell your doctors so they can help you avoid major health catastrophes.

If you are clueless about what to tell your health care providers, then it is hard for them to be of maximum service to you. Your personal involvement and awareness make all the difference in getting the best possible use of the health care you have access to and in making smart choices that can benefit your health now and in the future.

In consultation with your doctor and other appropriate health care providers, you can successfully chart a course for your health that makes sense and gets the results you are after. To improve the effectiveness of the time you spend with health professionals, this section focuses on what to ask the people who help you with your health and the risk factors for heart disease you need to be aware of.

Questions for You to Answer about Your Current Level of Heart Health

- Does heart disease in any form run in your family?
- If you don't have information on the health of your blood relatives, do you have any reason to suspect heart disease in any form ran in your family?

- Do you exercise regularly? Is your exercise primarily aerobic or anaerobic exercise?
- Do you know what role exercise, nutrition, stress management, fulfilling relationships, herbs, and supplements play in treating and preventing heart disease?
- What vitamins, herbs, homeopathic remedies, nutrients, and/or nutritional supplements do you take? Do you experience any side effects from them?
- Have you had any major life stresses in the past two years? (Some examples are a new job; loss of a job; moving more than 100 miles from your prior home; getting married; getting divorced; having more than one child under the age of three at home; death of a loved one; more debt than you can manage; or coping with life-threatening illness, either your own or someone else's.)
- If you take both pharmaceutical medicines and natural medicines or nutritional supplements, are there any interactions between them? What are those interactions and how could they affect you?
- Do you use a heart rate monitor to help you maximize the benefits of your exercise efforts?

Questions about Your Current Level of Heart Health for Your Doctor to Answer

- How much exercise is appropriate for you in the next month? Over the next three months?
- Should you seek the services of a personal trainer in formulating an exercise program tailored to you?
- What prescription medications do you take? Do you experience any side effects from them? How long do you need to take them and why?

Questions about Your Current Level of Heart Health for *You* and *Your Doctor* to Answer Together

- What is your entire health history? Are there any particular elements that may have special impact on heart disease, such as estrogen replacement therapy, diabetes, drinking alcohol, or smoking?

- If you have high blood pressure, is it affected by how much salt is in the food you eat?
- Is your strategy for managing stress effective, or do you need help?
- When was the last time you had a thorough physical exam? It should include a blood pressure check; pulse (heart rate) reading; someone listening carefully to your chest and heartbeat; reflexes check; eye exam; ears, nose, and throat exam; skin exam (especially moles or odd-appearing patches of skin); breast exam; Pap smear; and screening laboratory profiles using blood, saliva, stool, and/or urine. If it has been longer than a year, get an exam now. Do not delay.

Note: Encourage the African American men in your life to get a prostate exam in addition to the previous exams (except the Pap smear). This simple check can be life saving and a key part of prevention. In the United States, Black men have four times the incidence of prostate cancer and other disorders of the prostate, such as benign prostatic hypertrophy, as White men do.

Your Medical Records

Keep a copy of all your medical records, including lab test results and reports from specialists. This is valuable information concerning how your body functions. While you may not understand everything found in these types of records, it is extremely important that you maintain the information. If another health professional needs the information and you have it neatly arranged in a binder, in chronological order, this can be a huge help in speeding up key assessments concerning your health. Many health care offices are overwhelmed with paperwork, and requests for records can take time to fulfill. Also, since there is so much paper to manage in the medical setting, records do occasionally get lost or misfiled. Do yourself and your health care team a favor and keep all your records in one place, like a labeled binder, where you can quickly and easily find the information when it is needed.

Be sure you understand everything you are being tested for when your doctor runs lab work on your behalf. Ask questions so you can understand what is going on with your health. Keep copies of your lab work. If you do not feel comfortable asking questions or feel that you don't know what to say or how to say it, bring along a trusted friend to your appointments to help you get your questions answered. If your ability to concentrate or otherwise express yourself is not quite what you'd like, get the support of others who can be advocates for you. Your health care team is there to help you, and it is best if you let them know what you need and expect.

Resources

In this section, I list additional resources for your use—books, organizations, Web sites, and other places you can look for information, inspiration, and different points of view on the elements of great health. Some books listed here cover natural methods of health care, while others are quite steeped in conventional medicine. My goal is to stimulate your desire for great health and share with you as many resources as possible. If you ever feel confused by what appears to be conflicting or contradictory information, recognize that natural health and medicine are dynamic and evolving fields. Science is helping us to better understand the factors that influence us every day. Take it all under consideration and do what works for you. Remember, there is no such thing as one-size-fits-all health advice. May you enjoy your further health discoveries and find some treasures among the resources listed below. To your health!

Books

African American Health
Dixon, Barbara M., L.D.N., R.D., and Josleen Wilson. *Good Health for African Americans*. New York, NY: Crown Publishers, 1994.
Health and Healing for African Americans. Edited by Sheree Crute. Emmaus, PA: Rodale Press, 1997.

Behaviors of Wealth
Flores, Bettina, and Jennifer Basye Sander. *The Millionairess across the Street*. Dearborn, IL: Dearborn Financial Publishing, 1999.
Stanley, Thomas J., Ph.D., and William D. Danko, Ph.D. *The Millionaire*

Next Door: The Surprising Secrets of America's Wealthy. Marietta, GA: Longstreet Press, 1998.

Body & Soul: The Black Women's Guide to Physical Health and Emotional Well-Being. Edited by Linda Villarosa. New York, NY: HarperCollins Publishers, 1994.

Diabetes
Bernstein, Richard K., M.D., F.A.C.E. *Dr. Bernstein's Diabetes Solution: A Complete Guide to Achieving Normal Blood Sugars.* Boston, MA: Little, Brown and Co., 1997.

Fat and Its Role in Health
Erasmus, Udo. *Fats that Heal, Fats that Kill: The Complete Guide to Fats, Oils, Cholesterol, and Human Health.* Vancouver, BC: Alive Books, 1999.

Financial Planning and Wealth
Orman, Suze. *The 9 Steps to Financial Freedom.* New York, NY: Crown Publishers, 1997.
Orman, Suze. *The Courage to Be Rich: Creating a Life of Material and Spiritual Abundance.* New York, NY: Riverhead Books, 1999.
Orman, Suze, and Linda Mead. *You've Earned It, Don't Lose It: Mistakes You Can't Afford to Make When You Retire.* Revised and updated ed. New York, NY: Newmarket Press, 1998, 1999.

Herbs and Botanical Medicine
Grieve, Mrs. M. *A Modern Herbal.* Edited by Mrs. C. F. Leyel. 2 volumes. New York, NY: Dover Publications, 1971.

Natural Medicine
Murray, Michael, N.D., and Joseph Pizzorno, N.D. *Encyclopedia of Natural Medicine.* 2nd edition. Rocklin, CA: Prima Publishing, 1997.

Nutrition
D'Adamo, Dr. Peter, and Catherine Whitney. *Cook Right for Your Type.* New York, NY: G. P. Putnam's Sons, 1998.

D'Adamo, Dr. Peter, and Catherine Whitney. *Eat Right for Your Type*. New York, NY: G. P. Putnam's Sons, 1996.

Spiritual and Emotional Balance
Vanzant, Iyanla. *The Value in the Valley: A Black Woman's Guide through Life's Dilemmas*. New York, NY: Simon & Schuster, 1995.

Sports Performance
Douillard, John. *Body, Mind, and Sport: The Mind-Body Guide to Lifelong Fitness and Your Personal Best*. New York, NY: Crown Publishing, 1994.

Stress
Orioli, Esther. *StressMap: Personal Diary Edition*. New York, NY: New Market Press, 1991.

Weight Training
Phillips, Bill, and Michael D'Orso. *Body for Life*. New York, NY: HarperCollins Publishers, 1999.

Women's Health
Hudson, Tori, N.D. *Women's Encyclopedia of Natural Medicine: Alternative Therapies and Integrative Medicine*. Los Angeles, CA: Keats Publishing, 1999.
Love, Susan M., M.D., and Karen Lindsey. *Dr. Susan Love's Breast Book*. 2nd edition. Reading, MA: Addison-Wesley, 1995.
Love, Susan M., M.D., and Karen Lindsey. *Dr. Susan Love's Hormone Book*. New York, NY: Random House, 1997.

Internet Web Sites

www.naturalhealthcare.com
www.dryates.com (you can visit me on the Web)
www.drbeverlyyates.com (you can visit me on the Web here, too)

Professional Associations

Naturopathic Physicians
American Association of Naturopathic Physicians, 601 Valley St., Suite #105, Seattle, WA 98109; 206/298-0125. You can call to order a directory of licensed NDs for a nominal fee. The money pays for the cost of printing and mailing the directory. Web address is www.naturopathic.org.

Holistic Medical Doctors
American Holistic Medical Association (AHMA), 6728 Old McLean Village Dr., McLean, VA 22101; 703/556-9728; www.holisticmedicine.org

Massage Therapists
American Massage Therapy Association, 820 Davis St., Suite 100, Evanston, IL 60201; 847/864-0123; www.amtamassage.org

Acupuncturists and Traditional Chinese Medical Practitioners
National Certification Commission for Acupuncture and Oriental Medicine (NCCAOM), 11 Canal Center Plaza, Ste. 300, Alexandria, VA 22314; 703/548-9004; www.nccaom.org

This is How You Stay on Track for the Long Term

These checklists are provided to help you stay on track with your heart healthy habits. I recommend you use all of them for at least one year to assist you in your journey. The checklists can be used as milestones along the way, affiming what you are doing well and illuminating any areas that need reinforcement or change.

Daily Maintenance Checklists of Heart Healthy Activities

Post this list on your refrigerator or another place in your home where you will see it daily.

Today I did at least five of the following nine things for my present and future heart health:

_____ minimum 20 minutes aerobic exercise, with stretching before and after exercise

_____ nutrition—hearty and healthful

_____ stress management

_____ quiet time

_____ fun and play, laughter

_____ deep purposeful breathing

_____ prayer or meditation

_____ soothing music, healing sounds

_____ quality time to share my feelings and thoughts with loved ones

Meal checklists for quality of food eaten and quality of atmosphere in which it is eaten:

_____ Today I ate all of my meals at a relaxed pace and chewed my food thoroughly; I ate slowly enough that I was the last one to finish eating.

_____ All of the food I ate was truly nutritious.

_____ My food smelled good, tasted good, and looked good.

_____ The food I ate was high in fiber.

_____ I ate at least five servings today of fruits and vegetables.

_____ The food I ate was the highest quality I could get, preferably organic.

_____ The room I ate my food in was relaxing, calming, and free of conflict.

_____ My surroundings supported my sense of nourishment and nurturance on many levels.

_____ My breathing was even and my heart rate was slow during my meals.

Weekly "Formulas for Heart Health Success"

_____ I did aerobic exercise for 20 minutes or more at least four times this week.

_____ I spent time meditating or praying at least five times this week.

_____ I listened to enjoyable music or played a musical instrument at least three times this week.

_____ I ate a minimum of one meal each day that had excellent nutritional value. (This is seven or more great meals for the week.)

_____ I had two or more times this week where I spent genuine "heart connection" time with friends or family.

Monthly "Formulas for Heart Health Success"

_____ This month I took time just for myself at least once a week.

_____ I exercised 16 times or more this month.

_____ I ate at least 30 truly healthy meals this month.

_____ I finished a project that gave me relief when it was finished.

_____ I offered someone my help as a volunteer, or, I accepted someone's volunteer help.

_____ I had 25 percent or more fewer stressful moments this month than last month.

_____ I reached emotional closure on a challenging issue this month.

_____ I had two or more therapeutic, relaxing massages this month.

_____ I put in place whatever I needed to change to make it even easier and more likely that I will take excellent care of myself.

_____ I celebrated what I did right this month on behalf of my health.

Three-Month "Formulas for Heart Health Success"

_____ Have a blood pressure check at home, a clinic, or a pharmacy.

_____ Enjoy a weekend devoted to relaxation.

_____ Use two new heart healthy recipes for meals at home or on the go.

_____ Do a different type of aerobic exercise at least twice over three months.

_____ Take my resting pulse and notice if it is higher or lower than when I began my health program.

_____ Clean up old business in the emotional realm.

_____ Acknowledge and celebrate all the positive changes I've made in the last 90 days as well as all the good habits I already had.

Yearly "Formulas for Heart Health Success"

_____ I had a physical exam, including a blood pressure check and screening laboratory profiles using blood, saliva, stool and/or urine.

_____ I have two or more deepened, fulfilling relationships in my life.

_____ I used eight new heart healthy recipes for meals at home or on the go.

_____ I cut old emotional baggage by 50 percent or more during the year.

_____ I identified and eliminated any obstacles to excellent health.

_____ At least one week was devoted to rest, relaxation, and fun.

_____ I celebrated all the things I did right concerning my health.

_____'s Fun and Easy Exercise Checklist

Your Name Here

Make a list of physical activities you enjoy, such as skating, jumping rope, dancing, swimming, basketball, walking, etc.

Make two columns beside the list; label one column **FUN** and the other column **EASY**.

Place a number by each activity you wrote down, ranking them according to how much fun you have doing the activity. <u>Underline</u> the top 3 **fun** activities.

Now rank the activities according to how easy they are for you to do. <u>Highlight</u> the top three **easy** activities.

As you sort your list again, keep in mind the following criteria for "easy":

Does the activity require special equipment?

Do you need special clothes or access to a health club or pool?

Is the weather a factor in your being able to do the activity?

Do you need other people to do the exercise (for example, basketball, volleyball, or soccer)?

Do you have to travel to do the exercise (for example, skiing, snorkeling, scuba diving)?

Can you pop out of bed and begin the exercise in less than 15 minutes from waking up?

Are there any other limits, interfering factors, or considerations to your participation in this exercise?

Do you feel invigorated after your exercise routine, or do you feel sore, breathless, and exhausted? (If you feel wiped out, you are working too hard. Slow down.)

Remember to highlight the top three **easy** activities.

Circle the activity that appears on both the **FUN** list and the **EASY** list.

Make this activity that appears on both the **FUN** and the **EASY** lists the key exercise you do during weekdays—three to four times a week—at an aerobic pace.

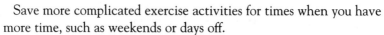

Save more complicated exercise activities for times when you have more time, such as weekends or days off.

Beware of making it either too hard or too complicated to exercise. Few people regularly do what is hard and complicated, especially if it relates to exercise.

Before you go to bed, lay out any clothing, shoes, or other equipment you need for your chosen exercise activity. This saves you time the next day and removes any procrastination that may be lurking about actually doing the exercise.

If appropriate, select your favorite music and play it while you exercise. This helps keep the fun level up! The music can help you stay in the aerobic range of exercise as you rhythmically move your body and limbs to the beat.

Celebrate your follow-through on your commitment to regular exercise with a *healthful* treat—several glasses of pure water, a cup of herbal tea, a massage, or some extra moments of quiet time.

Glossary

Amino Acid—essential building block of protein, used in repair of tissues, skin, gut, bones, etc.; certain illnesses respond well to specific amino acids

Arteries—blood vessels that take blood away from the heart and out to all the body's tissues

Botanical medicine—derived from plants considered to be medicinal herbs

Carbohydrate—basic unit of one of three broad categories of nutrition; too much promotes excessive release of insulin and can contribute to weight problems and diabetes; complex carbohydrates are preferred (unrefined whole grains and other complex carbohydrates are more healthful in general); too little can lead to constipation and slowed metabolism (nondiabetic)

Cardiovascular disease—diseases and illness that affects the heart or any of the blood vessels in the body

Cerebrovascular accident—medical name for stroke

Cholesterol—a kind of fat used by the body to make hormones (estrogen, progesterone, testosterone, etc.); serves as a multipurpose building block for various elements of health; often gets a bad reputation but is a necessary element of good health; what matters the most is what your body does with the cholesterol you have, especially how the liver processes cholesterol

Clot—clump of congealed blood and platelets

Coccidiomycosis—a fungal lung disease

Crash Diet—a mistake every time; it takes time to gain weight, it takes time to lose it and keep it off for good; this kind of diet often leaves the base metabolism too slow to maintain a healthful weight so the pounds steadily creep back on

Diet—a program of eating that hopefully achieves a specific result

Embolism—a blood clot that is moving or has moved from where it origi-nated in the body to a different location; often deadly because the clot can block major areas of blood flow, such as a lung or the brain

Essential Fatty Acid (EFA)—essential building block of healthful fats, must be present in the food you eat as your body cannot make this fat on its own; needed for normal nervous system function, healthy skin, gut, and hormonal balance

Estrogen—hormone found in much higher levels in women than in men, typically much lower after menopause; can be given as a prescription item; there are potential tradeoffs with its use—thought to be protective of the heart; however, excess estrogen can cause or contribute to breast, ovarian, and uterine cancers; best to be an informed consumer

Fad Diet—see Crash Diet

Fat—basic unit of one of three broad categories of nutrition; too much causes congestion of digestive functions, especially gall bladder (bile con-centration) and liver (bile production) functionality; too little can inter-fere with normal hormone, reproductive, and nervous system functions

Heart Attack—also known as myocardial infarction, occurs when the heart tissue itself does not get enough blood due to too little coronary blood circulation

Heart Disease—technically speaking, this is coronary artery disease (CAD); refers to blockage of the coronary arteries due to conditions that promote the accumulation of cholesterol along the arterial walls

Herb—a plant used for its ability to either promote wellness or help restore health; commonly spoken of in two ways, as culinary (cooking) herbs or as medicinal herbs

Homocysteine—a marker of cardiovascular and heart disease, it is toxic to arterial walls; levels can increase in women after menopause

Hormone—potent chemical made in the body by glands or organs for use in another part of the body

Insulin—hormone made in the pancreas that helps cells make use of the energy found in glucose (blood sugar); body's premiere fat-building and fat-storage hormone; balanced levels promote normal, healthful weight range

Menopause—time when the menstrual cycle stops; technically, it is the time of the last menstrual period

Metabolism—rate at which the body burns fuel for energy

Mineral—chemical whose properties as an electrolyte help provide the "spark" to numerous bodily processes; critical for proper heart function, nervous system balance, immune function, and muscular performance

Nutrition—balanced blend of healthful foods in proportions that make sense for you, eaten at intervals that work for your metabolism

Perimenopause—transitional time before menopause when the menstrual cycle is about to stop; common for the menses to speed up, slow down, or exhibit other changes before it stops all together

Phlebitis—inflammation of the veins

Phytonutrients—nutrients found in plants that are known to have medicinal or healthful properties

Platelets—nature's Band-Aids™; in a normal response to injury, platelets are needed to help wounds heal properly

Progesterone—hormone found in much higher levels in women than in men, typically much lower after menopause; can be given as a prescription item; there are potential tradeoffs with its use; often prescribed with estrogen to help balance the effects of estrogen (see Estrogen); best to be an informed consumer

Protein—basic unit of one of three broad categories of nutrition; too much causes a person to lose minerals from their bones and overworks the kidneys in excreting the by-products of processing the protein; too little makes it hard for body to do basic repair, especially of muscle and intestinal/digestive tissues

Slavery—in this book refers to period of New World history (1400s–1865) when Africans were sold into slavery by other Africans to Europeans and transported to North America, the Caribbean, Central, and South America

Starch—also known as carbohydrate

Stroke—occurs either when there is a blockage of blood flow to the affected tissue or when blood leaks into tissue inappropriately (the brain is a common site)

Sugar—simple carbohydrate, causes insulin and adrenal function to go on a roller coaster, which is not healthful; very little good to be said about sugar

Thromboses—medical name for clots, which are excessive accumulation of sticky platelets

Transient ischemic attacks (TIAs)—temporary lack of blood flow to a bodily tissue, typically the brain is the affected tissue. Usually, TIAs do not result in permanent damage to the affected tissue.

Varicose veins—these are veins that have lost much of their structural integrity; as a result, they can become the site(s) of clots, phlebitis, or embolisms; tend to be hereditary

Varicosities—multiple locations of varicose veins

Veins—blood vessels that return blood from all the body's tissues to the lungs where it will be reoxygenated

Vitamin—essential nutrient found in food that is used by the body to create and maintain health

Notes

Use these pages to record your thoughts and progress. These pages are for you.

Notes

Notes

Notes

Index

About the Author

Author and board certified naturo-pathic physician, Dr. Beverly Yates, was born and raised in Philadelphia, Pennsylvania. As a naturopathic physician, Dr. Yates thrives on the interaction she gets with her patients. She finds the rewarding process of seeking the most effective natural therapies for each individual much like fitting the pieces of a puzzle together.

A graduate of both the National College of Naturopathic Medicine and Massachusetts Institute of Technology, Dr. Yates has presented

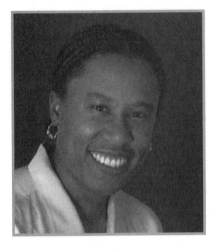

Dr. Beverly Yates

seminars about natural health care to audiences across the country. Dr. Yates has additional training as a licensed massage therapist and in proc-tological procedures, emergency medicine, outpatient surgery, and critical care procedures. Dr. Yates is a member of the American Association of Naturopathic Physicians (AANP) and the Occidental Research Institute Foundation. She's board certified to practice naturopathy in Hawaii, Oregon, and Washington; however, she currently practices and makes her home in Seattle, Washington.

For more information about Dr. Yates or heart health for Black women, see her Web sites: www.dryates.com, www.drbeverlyyates.com, or www.naturalhealthcare.com.